W9-DIT-974

Disease, medicine and society in England, 1550–1860

Second Edition

New Studies in Economic and Social History

Edited for the Economic History Society by
Michael Sanderson
University of East Anglia, Norwich

This series, specially commissioned by the Economic History Society, provides a guide to the current interpretations of the key themes of economic and social history in which advances have recently been made or in which there has been significant debate.

In recent times economic and social history has been one of the most flourishing areas of historical study. This has mirrored the increasing relevance of the economic and social sciences both in a student's choice of career and in forming a society at large more aware of the importance of these issues in their everyday lives. Moreover specialist interests in business, agricultural and welfare history, for example, have themselves burgeoned and there has been an increased interest in the economic development of the wider world. Stimulating as these scholarly developments have been for the specialist, the rapid advance of the subject and the quantity of new publications make it difficult for the reader to gain an overview of particular topics, let alone the whole field.

New Studies in Economic and Social History is intended for students and their teachers. It is designed to introduce them to fresh topics and to enable them to keep abreast of recent writing and debates. All the books in the series are written by a recognised authority in the subject, and the arguments and issues are set out in a critical but unpartisan fashion. The aim of the series is to survey the current state of scholarship, rather than to provide a set of prepackaged conclusions.

The series has been edited since its inception in 1968 by Professors M. W. Flinn, T. C. Smout and L. A. Clarkson, and is currently edited by Dr Michael Sanderson. From 1968 it was published by Macmillan as *Studies in Economic History*, and after 1974 as *Studies in Economic and Social History*. From 1995 *New Studies in Economic and Social History* is being published on behalf of the Economic History Society by Cambridge University Press. This new series includes some of the titles previously published by Macmillan as well as new titles, and reflects the ongoing development throughout the world of this rich seam of history.

For a full list of titles in print, please see the end of the book.

Disease, medicine and society in England, 1550–1860

Second Edition

Prepared for the Economic History Society by

Roy Porter
Wellcome Institute for the History of Medicine, London

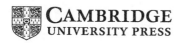

CAMBRIDGE
UNIVERSITY PRESS

285 215

SEP 10 2003

Published by the Press Syndicate of the University of Cambridge
The Pitt Building, Trumpington Street, Cambridge CB2 1RP
40 West 20th Street, New York, NY 10011-4211, USA
10 Stamford Road, Oakleigh, Melbourne 3166, Australia

Disease, Medicine and Society in England, 1550–1860 was published by The
Macmillan Press Limited 1987
Second edition published by The Macmillan Press Limited 1993
First Cambridge University Press edition 1995

Printed in Great Britain at the University Press, Cambridge

A catalogue record for this book is available from the British Library

Library of Congress cataloguing in publication data

ISBN 0 521 55262 1 hardback
ISBN 0 521 55791 7 paperback

CE

Contents

Introduction to the second edition   *page* vii

Introduction   1

1   Disease, death and doctors in Tudor and
    Stuart England   5

2   The practice of medicine in early modern
    England   11

3   Experiences and actions: countering illness in
    the seventeenth and eighteenth centuries   17

4   Medicine in the market economy of the
    Georgian age   27

5   The medical profession and the state in the
    nineteenth century   45

6   The role of medicine: what did it achieve?   59

Select bibliography   64
Index   77

Introduction to the second edition

This brief book was written in 1986. Seven years later, I am delighted that there is a demand for a second edition. I am even more pleased that, in the meantime, a large quantity of high-quality research and synthetic writing has appeared on the history of British health and medicine between the sixteenth and the nineteenth centuries. To accommodate this new work, in this second edition I have considerably revised the text, both in regard to details and in its wider views. I have also updated and extended the bibliography. I trust this book now represents a synthesis of our present understanding of the age.

A note on references

References in the text within square brackets relate to the numbered items in the Select Bibliography.

A note on language

To avoid clumsiness, I have, in the traditional manner, used the male pronouns (he, his) in the generic sense. When referring to regular doctors, my use of the pronoun 'he' is always literally accurate, since in the period covered by this book, only males could become practitioners. In Britain, women were debarred from the medical profession till the 1870s.

Introduction

From a social history viewpoint, this book examines the impact of disease upon English people, and responses to sickness, lay and medical alike. Its chronology, roughly 1550–1860, spans early modern times and the first century of industrial society; this allows questions to be asked both about enduring traditions and about change – for instance, the impact of rapid urbanisation upon the people's health [120]. It broaches certain issues that are primarily demographic, by asking what part disease and medicine played in bringing about adjustments in population levels and profiles. It touches upon socioeconomic history, by examining the wealth and professional power of medical practitioners. And it asks some questions germane to the administrative or political historian: what role did the state play in promoting public health? But it is not chiefly any of these – nor is it a reassessment of the roots of the welfare state or of the National Health Service [109; 124]. Its main concern lies rather with responses – social, religious and medical alike – to sickness and to threats of death. Central to that story is an assessment of changing relations between the people at large and the medical profession.

In its organisation, this pamphlet attempts to combine thematic and chronological approaches. The first chapter briefly sketches the 'biological *ancien régime*' as it affected English society between Tudor times and the surge of industrialisation. How severe were the threats disease posed to the population at large and to the social fabric? Did medicine offer any real defences against disease? Chapter 2 then focuses upon the social presence of medicine in pre-industrial England. How was healing practised and who practised it? Were there many grass roots 'healers'? Was medicine largely the preserve of professional doctors, or did it lie in the hands of the people as well? Looking from the inside, Chapter 3 explores this world of short lives and sudden death. What did it feel like to live in times when health and existence itself were both utterly precarious? How did the sick evaluate doctors and the services they offered? How far did people try medical self-help? Or were they fatalistic, resigned to their fate and to the will of God? Attention is briefly given to seventeenth- and eighteenth-century attitudes, but these persisted well into the nineteenth century.

The fourth chapter examines in greater detail the development of the medical profession from the eighteenth century. Who were the doctors? What social rank did they enjoy? How many were there? What types of practitioners were there, on a spectrum ranging from the orthodox, through the irregular, to the shameless quack? How well did practitioners meet demands for medical services in a commercialized economy increasingly geared to the free market and to 'consumerism', that is, the provision of goods and services in return for cash payment [4]?

If Chapter 4 examines the private relations of doctors to their clients in bedside medicine, Chapter 5 proceeds to consider practitioners in their collective and public roles, particularly in the nineteenth century. How did the many distinct, and frequently competing, types of practitioner comprising medicine as a whole relate to each other? How was medicine able to consolidate itself as a prestigious profession, rather than remaining just another 'white-collar' occupation like school-teaching or journalism? The answers to these questions are obviously connected with the growing employment of medical men by the Victorian state as part of its new commitment to public health. The effects of medicine's entry onto the public stage will be assessed.

In terms of preserving 'endangered lives' [138], what did all this medical activity amount to? Could the rise of the medical profession, linked to a new 'scientific medicine' and the 'sanitary science' of the public health movement, achieve much to reduce morbidity and mortality? Were English people healthier in 1850 than in 1750, 1650 or 1550? Were they living longer? And if so, how far was that thanks to medicine? Such issues are tackled in Chapter 6 [107]. An important problem emerges: if, even in the mid-nineteenth century, medicine was still not especially successful in preserving health and conquering disease, how do we explain the growing presence and prestige of the medical profession amongst the Victorians?

Fierce debates have raged between rival schools of historians as to how to interpret the march of medicine from Victorian times that culminated in the National Health Service, inaugurated in 1948. Doctors have generally stressed the part played by advances in medical science: scientific medicine has packed increasing curative power. Historians by contrast tend to stress the importance of reform, humanitarianism and state intervention. By contrast, radical, feminist and Marxist scholars have recently offered revisionist interpretations of a more sombre cast: in the eyes of some, the rise of modern medicine should be regarded as a saga of professional aggrandisement, monopoly, profiteering and of the use (or abuse) of medical power to enhance 'social control'. Debate has been lively on these issues. Feminist scholars have argued, for instance, that medical diagnoses like hysteria were widely used to keep women in their place by showing they were weak and sick [32]. Edward Shorter by contrast has implied that women's emancipation owes more to medicine than to the Suffragettes [116].

The generalisations presented below rest upon contested and sometimes shaky evidence. Partly this is because vast areas still remain to be researched. Thus only a few in-depth studies have been made of the functioning of hospitals within industrialising communities [90; 108] or of the workings of lunatic asylums [29]. The dangers of generalising from a few cases are obvious. But partly the problem is that the past is all too often silent: essential evidence simply has not survived. Thus it is highly probable that large numbers of female healers (so-called 'wise women') possessed valuable medical skills in traditional society: indeed, some feminists have claimed that 'witches' fulfilled important medical roles [32]. Unfortunately, whereas a fair number of autobiographies and case-books of male practitioners survive, we lack equivalents from female healers [48]. Their outlooks and practices must be deduced second or third hand, often from highly hostile sources. Uneven survival of documentary evidence and the biases of scholars mean that we currently know less about lay medicine than professional, less about irregular than about official therapies, less about women than men. That does not mean that the former in each pair were not important. Not least, though it is important to look 'from below', the lower we look down the social scale, the less the information, and the less satisfactory it is [94]. Moreover, despite the heroic efforts of historical demographers, all attempts to provide statistical profiles of life chances before the first census in 1801 are necessarily tentative [141].

This survey covers England, not Britain as a whole. It says nothing about Ireland and Wales, and not much about health care and medicine in Scotland [45], or, for that matter, the expanding British Empire [27]. These regrettable gaps mirror the uneven state of current research. Here and there, however, a contrast with Continental Europe or America has been introduced, to highlight distinctive features of English medicine [103; 122]. Little is said below either about epidemiology, or about the progress of medical science as such. For these McGrew [71] provides a clear and comprehensive reference work. For longer time-spans and more international perspectives, see [14], while for lucid narratives of medicine and society see [127; 135; 136].

1
Disease, death and doctors in Tudor and Stuart England

Radical Puritans in the English Revolution (1642–60) wanted to transform the nation's institutions 'root and branch'. Not least amongst the evils they abhorred and aimed to eradicate was the existing medical profession. Reformers such as William Dell maintained that healing had been perverted by the corrupt, privileged clique who controlled London's Royal College of Physicians (chartered in 1518), and thereby regulated other practitioners. This learned elite, academically trained in Greek medicine through a protracted university education, dogmatically upheld (so reformers alleged) the exploded medical system associated with the authority of the Graeco-Roman physician Galen and other 'ancients'. By using the powers granted to it by royal charter to restrict membership and thereby to police London medical practice, the College oligarchy, bent on power and profit, was, the radicals claimed, blocking the spread of newer, better approaches to healing, in particular that identified with the Swiss reformer Paracelsus, which was more popular and open, and favoured simpler, cheaper drug remedies [39; 133]. Physicians, complained the religious radical, Lodowick Muggleton, were 'the greatest cheats in the world' [126].

In critics' eyes, the universities and medical colleges had conspired to pervert English medicine, so that it provided unlimited (though largely worthless) treatment for the rich and all too little for the rest. Radicals proposed numerous schemes for reorganisation. They vowed to make medical education, knowledge and practice far more open, above all by replacing Latin with English as the language of the profession. Some proposed state-funded 'research centres' for the advancement of medical science along the lines advocated by Francis Bacon. And they urged public provision of free or cheap medical facilities, including hospitals for the sick poor, proposing plans that dimly anticipated the National Health Service [133].

Puritans were right to think that English medicine had little reason to be proud of itself. The shortcomings of Oxford and Cambridge in providing medical education were underscored by the fact that nearly all top English physicians had studied abroad, mainly in France and Italy. In any case, only a small percentage of medical practitioners had actually attended university, and those learned, gentlemanly physicians clustered in London, where the Court, City and Parliament provided the highest concentration of prosperous patients and so the richest pickings. Outside London, academically-trained doctors formed but a small minority; thus five out of seventy-five practitioners known to have operated between 1570 and 1590 in Norwich – then England's second largest city – had been to university [132]. Most practitioners had gained their skills as surgeons or apothecaries (roughly equal to today's dispensing chemists) by apprenticeship. They had no formal anatomical or scientific training.

Above all, critics denied that traditional medicine as taught in the universities did much good. The prating, pompous physician, spouting Greek aphorisms, was an easy satirical target; and the experiences of the decimating waves of influenza and 'the sweat' in mid-Tudor times, or the dreadful epidemics that devastated the Stuart age – in particular, the successive outbreaks of plague, culminating in the carnage of 1665 – did nothing to enhance doctors' reputations [119]. It did not help, for instance, that most fellows of the College of Physicians fled London during the 1665 plague outbreak, or that the royal physicians made such a botch of the final illness of Charles II.

Worse still, medicine plainly had no answers to the fatal diseases that time and again proved such scourges. Across Europe, the seventeenth century saw a marked deterioration in the climate, poor harvests, frequent dearth and chronic malnutrition caused by excessive population pressure upon economic resources. Against this background, epidemics of various fevers and infectious diseases, including smallpox and, most terrifyingly, bubonic plague, struck and struck again, checking the population rise that had formed such a conspicuous feature of the Tudor century. In early Stuart England, the life expectation was probably under thirty-five years [19; 25]. Infants and children were particularly vulnerable. The great diarist, Samuel Pepys, had ten brothers and sisters: only two survived into adulthood. Many factors combined to make the population vulnerable: poverty, dearth, overwork, repeated pregnancies (there was no contraception in the modern sense), insanitary and overcrowded living conditions. But in England – contrary to the experience of many parts of Europe – it was disease rather than famine that actually proved a killer [2].

And against such diseases, the healer's art proved a broken reed. The strengths and weaknesses of 'learned medicine' for those who could afford it remained those of the medicine of Antiquity, particularly that of Hippocrates and Galen, on whose authority it leant so heavily. Orthodox medicine set great store by the management of a healthy life through regulation of diet, exercise and the pursuit of moderation. It also prided itself upon its clinical perceptiveness, bred of centuries of experience. But its powers to combat disease had advanced very little since the Ancients. The emphasis of its therapeutics lay on expelling toxic substances from the body – by purging, sweating, vomiting and the much-favoured surgical technique of bloodletting (see cover illustration). It aimed to restore 'balance', and to fortify the body's regular constitution. To these ends, scores of medicaments might be used. Tried and trusted simple herbal preparations had long been augmented by complex and often very expensive drugs, such as 'theriac', compounded of dozens of exotic ingredients, many deriving from Arab medicine. Certain chemical, mineral and metallic ingredients, like antimony and mercury – advocated for venereal conditions by the sixteenth-century medical iconoclast, Paracelsus – were also being introduced into the drug repertoire. Many of these preparations 'worked', in the sense that they brought about a predicted and visible effect: they did indeed cause purging and vomiting. But very few of the recipes that physicians prescribed and apothecaries dispensed 'worked' in the sense that, say, antibiotics work, that is by destroying the micro-organisms which caused people to die from diphtheria, pneumonia, typhus and a multitude of other infections. These bacteria were as yet totally unknown.

It was basic research (in biology, chemistry, bacteriology and immunology) that would eventually enable late-nineteenth and twentieth-century medicine to combat micro-organisms and sepsis. Seventeenth-century doctors lacked that science. Neither did early pharmacology prove very successful in coming up with 'wonder drugs' or even very effective pain-killers. Paracelsus had advocated mercury as a specific cure for syphilis, that new scourge introduced into Europe, probably from the New World, at the end of the fifteenth century – and mercury had proved reasonably effective, if highly unpleasant. Otherwise the drugs front was not very encouraging. Jesuits' Bark (or Peruvian Bark, a product of the cinchona tree, and the basis of quinine) was effective against malaria (the 'ague'), still endemic in low-lying areas like Romney Marsh; but it was little used before the latter part of the seventeenth century. And the same applies to opium, powerful as a pain-killer, a sedative and valuable for stopping dysentery and soothing coughs.

Traditional surgery could offer little more. Surgeons performed a multitude of useful items of 'external medicine', dressing wounds, manipulating dislocations, lancing boils, pulling teeth and, not least, letting blood, though in the days before the need for scrupulous cleanliness was understood, even these routine treatments, if performed with dirty hands and tainted instruments, might prove hazardous. Surgeons also set broken bones, dreadfully common mishaps in a work-world in which almost all power was manpower and in which travel by horse on rutted roads or cross-country meant high casualty figures. Experience had taught, however, that all but the most simple breaks turned septic or gangrenous. Hence, faced with a compound fracture of the leg or arm, surgeons would generally amputate – again a hazardous business, and a nightmare ordeal for the sufferer in days before the introduction of anaesthetics.

Unlike today's surgeon, however, his seventeenth-century fore-bear undertook little internal surgery (it was too dangerous and painful). Surgeons like the London practitioner, Joseph Binns, tended to be cautious [3]. Disorders of the heart, liver, brain or stomach were treated not by the surgeon's knife but by medicines and management. Brave folks like Pepys would submit to the knife for the common complaint of a bladder stone rather than endure a lifetime's excruciating pain: luckily for him and for us, the diarist was one of the fortunate ones who survived unscathed [94]. But major internal surgery was not feasible before the introduction of anaesthetics and antiseptic procedures in the mid-nineteenth century. Very occasionally, a surgeon would cut open a woman dying in labour to deliver a baby that could not be born naturally, but there is no record of any Englishwoman surviving a Caesarian section till the close of the eighteenth century [30; 116]. In general, the only bodies surgeons were accustomed to cutting open were dead ones, for post mortems and anatomical instruction; but in Britain, dissection long remained rare [105].

In other words, in early modern times, medicine was still losing the war against disease. Nowadays, when we fall sick, we expect medicine to cure or at least relieve us, and with good reason. Not so, three or four hundred years ago. This is not to say that people always despaired of the doctor and spurned his medicines. Medical men (and women healers) were clearly in demand. Neither were all measures against disease hopeless. As Slack's studies of plague have proved, energetic measures were commonly taken – more so in the seventeenth than in the sixteenth century – to halt the spread of the pestilence; travel and trade were restricted, stricken families were strictly quarantined within their own homes, domestic animals were destroyed, infected buildings were fumigated [118; 119]. Such central and local government ordinances might in limited ways be effective. The stringent precautions enforced by Thomas Wentworth, President of the Council of the North, in 1631 to protect York – he isolated the city and demolished the squalid shanty-town suburbs outside the city tenanted by the poor – perhaps explain why that city escaped pestilence whereas others like Bristol and Hull succumbed. Yet the effective measures were administrative and policing actions rather than medical cures – thereby in some ways anticipating the claim made by many nineteenth-century sanitary reformers that politicians could do more for public health than physicians. Despite these efforts, however, it remains clear that early modern medicine had no real answers to the epidemics that might easily sweep away a tenth of the inhabitants of a village within a year, or to the stomach and bowel disorders that killed off perhaps a third of new-born babies, toddlers and children under the age of five. Nowadays most people die old. Three hundred years ago, infections and constitutional disorders routinely killed people in the prime of life: teenagers, women in child-bed, and bread-winners.

Vulnerable to criticism, orthodox medicine had critics aplenty: alternative healers, satirists, fundamentalist preachers (who condemned it all as vanity: the cure of souls not of bodies was what counted), and those Puritan reformers mentioned earlier with their blueprints of public medicine for all. Despite all the criticism, almost nothing was achieved. The Puritan Revolution came and went without restructuring, redistributing or augmenting medical provision in England.

2

The practice of medicine in early modern England

When people fell sick in pre-industrial England, what medical facilities were available for them [132]? Well-off city-dwellers had access to an integrated pyramid of practitioners. At the top was the physician, whose job was to diagnose the complaint, make a prognosis of likely developments, prescribe treatments and medicines (which the apothecary would then dispense), and provide attendance and advice. 'Physic' called itself a liberal profession, founded upon a superior, university education. Physicians serving the social elite were expected to have a genteel demeanour to match that of their patients. Top physicians crowded into the capital, where fellows and licentiates of the Royal College of Physicians enjoyed by charter a monopoly of practice [17]. Around 1600, London physicians numbered nearly fifty, and in the seventeenth century the College jealously and zealously upheld its privileges through the law courts. Beyond the metropolis, a sprinkling of physicians practised in corporate towns, cathedral cities and wherever a better class of patients could be found. At least eleven physicians practised in Norwich between 1570 and 1590, six of them academically trained. Outside the cities, distribution of university-educated physicians was scanty, though many claimed to practise 'physic'.

Humbler in status than the physician was the surgeon. His was a manual craft rather than an intellectual science, involving the hand not the head. His job – very occasionally, *hers*, for there were a few female surgeons – was to treat external complaints (skin conditions, boils, wounds, injuries and so forth), to set bones and perform simple operations. Because both were arts of the knife, surgery and barbering had long been yoked together within the guild system, the Barber Surgeons Company of London dating from 1540; the two trades did not divorce and go their separate ways till 1745 [23]. The formal entry qualification for admission into the London Company, or into its equivalents in other corporate towns, lay in serving an indentured apprenticeship, normally for a period of seven years.

Beneath the surgeon in the medical pecking-order was the apothecary or druggist. Within the profession, the apothecary's status was lowly because he kept shop and pursued trade; his education was the 'mechanical' one of apprenticeship rather than the liberal one of the university. The apothecary was the physician's underling. The physician prescribed, the apothecary dispensed the prescription. Naturally there was great scope for rivalry between the two branches; knowing more than physicians about drugs, apothecaries often sought to prescribe on their own authority (clients were glad of this, since it eliminated the physician's hefty fee). In London this rivalry led to friction and legal wrangling between the College of Physicians and the Worshipful Society of Apothecaries, founded in 1617 and legally subject to supervision from the College [14; 24]. Through the seventeenth century the College of Physicians generally managed to uphold its rights, though at the cost of some loss of public sympathy. Outside London, however, such demarcation disputes were rare, for they flared up only where different grades of practitioners were independently incorporated and were treading on each other's toes. In Norwich, for instance, surgeons and physicians were organised in one and the same guild [132]. In small market towns, villages, and in the countryside, there was generally just a single practitioner (if that!) to a particular area, who would turn his hand to all types of healing, no matter what his formal training or name. Increasingly, in the eighteenth century, 'surgeon apothecary' was the title most commonly given to the country or small-town practitioner (whether he had been trained and qualified in both or not), signalling the indisputable need for the doctor to practise all aspects of medicine. In all but name, he had already become the general practitioner or family doctor [6; 69].

We do not as yet know how many regularly-trained practitioners were at work in Tudor or Stuart England. The first national 'medical register', published in 1779 and 1783, lists about 3000 (the total must have been somewhat higher) [63]. It is likely that numbers were rising during the eighteenth century, though we should not automatically assume that doctors were in short supply in Tudor and Stuart times. Painstaking research by Webster and Pelling has uncovered impressive numbers of early practitioners. In the London of Shakespeare's day, some 50 physicians, 100 surgeons, 100 apothecaries and 250 additional 'irregulars' were practising, to say nothing of midwives and nurses. Provincial towns might be similarly well-stocked. The names are known of almost a hundred practitioners active in Norwich between 1550 and 1600 [132]. Rural areas, however, were almost certainly much more poorly served than the towns. It might be symptomatic, for example, that the Revd Ralph Josselin, vicar of Earl's Colne in rural Essex, who kept an exceptionally full diary between the years 1643 and 1683, almost never called in a physician or a surgeon despite the endless stream of ailments and accidents suffered by him and his family [93].

Even where regular doctors were few and far between, there was never any shortage of other people experienced in caring for the sick. Such 'empirics' or 'irregulars' came in many guises. Some practised full-time, others once in a while; some for money, others out of charity; some were licensed, most were tolerated, a few were prosecuted. Amongst recognised practitioners were authorised midwives (all female). Midwives required a licence from the local bishop which principally testified to the woman's character. Good morals and religious soundness rather than medical skill were the official criteria of fitness to attend births, because midwives so easily fell under suspicion of dabbling in abortion and conniving at the infanticide of bastard babies (though there is little sign that they were widely suspected of witchcraft). The competence of traditional midwives is a matter of historical dispute. The male 'accoucheurs' – or obstetricians – who supplanted them in polite society during the eighteenth century represented the traditional 'granny midwife' as ignorant and inept. Recent research has shown, however, that many midwives were literate and came from respectable families. They probably managed normal deliveries well, though they may have lacked the expertise, practice and instruments needed to cope with the exceptional and tricky birth [9; 30; 116].

Another type of medical practitioner who might possess the legal protection of a licence was, paradoxically, the street-corner quack or 'empiric'. Mountebanks, mainly from France and Italy, could purchase royal privileges to practise, just as 'empirics' (practitioners with no formal training) could patent their 'nostrums' and proprietary medicines. Ever pinched for funds, Stuart monarchs were glad of the income derived from selling these rights, although the medical top-brass found it a scandal. In any case, the Stuarts had a stake of their own in irregular healing, since it was their practice to 'touch for the king's evil' (that is, the glandular disorder, scrofula): in 1712 the young Samuel Johnson was to be one of the last children so 'touched' [10].

Thousands of other people at this time made a living, or topped up their income, from medicine. Grocers and pedlars sold drugs. Blacksmiths and farriers drew teeth and set bones, doubling in human and veterinary medicine. Itinerants toured the country, selling bottles of brightly-coloured 'wonder cures' and moving on to the next town fast. Some were probably utter rogues like the mountebank in Ben Jonson's *Volpone*. Other travelling doctors possessed genuine skills in treating eye, teeth or ear complaints, thus performing a useful service in the days before business was brisk enough to support permanent, resident opticians or dentists in country towns.

Far more people, however, practised healing without any view to reward, but out of motives of neighbourliness, paternalism, good housekeeping, Christian charity or simple self-help. Every village had its nurses and 'wise women' well-versed in herb-lore and in secret brews and potions, their medicine often blending into white magic and sometimes verging on black. The gentry and clergy prided themselves upon their knowledge of physic, and treated their servants, households and parishioners as a matter of piety, duty and dire necessity. Their wives would also play 'lady bountiful' to the sick. As surviving manuscripts and printed recipe books show, skills in home-made medicines formed as much a part of good housewifery for a lady as making her own soap, beer and preserves out of the produce of the kitchen garden, woods and hedgerows [93].

Some went beyond this, and claimed special healing gifts. For instance, the Irish gentleman, Valentine Greatrakes, discovered he could cure through laying on of hands. His fame spread, and he came to England, holding healing sessions even at the court of Charles II, to the consternation of jealous physicians and scientists alike. One distinguishing feature of the 'free spirit' religious sects flourishing during the Civil War and Interregnum was faith-healing. George Fox, founder of the Quakers, even expected to raise people from the dead.

'Lay' medicine was sometimes attacked by regular practitioners. But it was almost all perfectly legal; only irregulars who brazenly trespassed upon the privileges of the London Colleges and Companies or the provincial guilds, found themselves indicted before the courts. And it filled a gap for those who could not afford regular practitioners, those who lived too far from them, those who had tried regular medicine to no avail, and, not least, those who distrusted putting their lives in doctors' hands and who thought, by analogy with radical Protestantism, that every man should be his own physician.

Thus, although there were probably fewer professional doctors in Tudor and Stuart times than in later centuries, the presence of a mixed bag of popular healers meant that few needing medical attention would have gone without. And that includes even the very poor. For physicians and quacks alike often made a point of treating some poor patients gratis, out of charity [85]. Moreover, institutional philanthropy also helped the sick poor. The Reformation under Henry VIII and Edward VI had certainly destroyed most charities designed to give refuge and medical care to the sick, the old and the infirm. In London, few institutions of medical consequence had survived the Reformation except St Thomas's Hospital, St Bartholomew's Hospital, and Bethlem Hospital (popularly called Bedlam: long England's only public madhouse). By European standards, seventeenth-century England was exceptionally ill-endowed with hospitals or plague-houses, or with sister institutions such as orphanages. Yet research is now revealing that more small almshouses and hospices were being founded by charitable bequests in Tudor and Stuart times than has generally been thought.

Moreover, within the framework of the Elizabethan Poor Law, modified at the Restoration of Charles II, parish paternalism frequently involved no small outlay of ratepayers' money on the sick or infirm, out of a mixture of genuine neighbourliness and enlightened self-interest. The sick and the mentally ill were commonly committed to the nursing care of other poor parishioners. Medicines, foods and funerals would be provided, and doctors' fees reimbursed for treating the poor. In the eighteenth century it became common for parishes to contract with a particular general practitioner to treat paupers for a fixed annual sum. Sometimes the amounts laid out on individuals appear surprisingly generous. It was not unknown to pay to send a sick person to a spa or to London for treatment, doubtless hoping that such outlays would, in the long run, prove cheaper than the cost of lifelong parish relief. Pauper hospitals were a rarity under the Old Poor Law (Bristol pioneered the pauper hospital, as it pioneered the workhouse) [35]; but in the days before friendly societies, charity and Poor Law relief combined to offer at least some medical attention to the lower orders [86; 123; 125].

3

Experiences and actions: countering illness in the seventeenth and eighteenth centuries

People of every age-group, occupation and social rank in early modern England knew they trod the pilgrim's progress of life in the shadow of sickness, disability and death. As they walked through the churchyard on Sunday or listened to the preacher, adults felt all around them the massive evidence of death: tombstones commemorating their grandparents, one or both parents, brothers and sisters who had died in infancy, and not least their own children. Youngsters might grow up wearing the clothes of dead siblings, and it was not uncommon for the newest born to be given the name of an already deceased brother or sister. Christianity itself hinged upon the great mystery of death; funerals were celebrated with infinitely more pomp than marriages or baptisms, and new secular cultural forms also accorded great prominence to mortality, not least newspaper obituary columns [41; 66].

Illness and death loomed large in people's minds. This is amply confirmed by the age's sermons and works of religious comfort, and above all through examination of the fragmentary remains left by individuals in commonplace books, journals, letters and diaries [93]. Such sources are of course socially unrepresentative – they record the thoughts of a minority of exceptional, literate people in a society in which a majority were illiterate. At least before the eighteenth century, our first-hand evidence from women is scanty, and such documents give almost no insight into the minds of children. But letters and diaries do tell us much. Their writers regularly take note of deaths in the community. Illness is a constant theme – that of the diarists themselves, their family and friends. What is more, such documents offer a window onto a wider 'sickness culture', revealing beliefs about the meanings of life and death, about the causes and purposes of sickness, about prevention and cure, about the relations between body and soul, flesh and spirit. For the early modern mentality, the condition of the body, registering as it did the ups and downs of health and sickness, meshed with wider perceptions of social, moral and spiritual well-being, of identity and destiny.

Furthermore, personal preoccupations with sickness, found in letter-writers and diarists like Samuel Pepys and the Puritan Richard Baxter, mirrored larger concerns. Remedies against sickness, omens foreshadowing dying, consolations for sufferers: these mattered in a popular culture passed down orally, almost literally with one's mother's milk; but they were also intoned from the pulpit, read in the Bible and similar religious works, and even picked up from the printed health-care manuals, like William Buchan's *Domestic Medicine* (1769), that first started appearing in Tudor times and had become extremely popular by the nineteenth century [93; 99; 132].

It would be naive to assume that people believed every word that doctors told them about medicine or all that preachers thundered about the corruption of the flesh. Contemporary diaries record how writers often ignored their doctors' advice. They did not always follow the recommendations they heard or read (how many people nowadays avidly read health-care columns and continue to smoke or over-eat!). But there was clearly some concurrence between public opinion and private experiences: and this allows us, however, tentatively, to piece together the 'sickness culture' of the centuries before the Industrial Revolution and previous to the emergence of modern, scientific medicine.

To do this, it may first be helpful to contrast this older health lore with assumptions widespread today. For most people nowadays, good health is a normal expectation, sickness an annoying and temporary interruption to a lengthy span of vigorous activity, maybe well over seventy years, whose termination seems remote enough to be safely put out of mind. Disease is thus seen as an exceptional intrusion. Falling ill can generally be explained (following popular understanding of Pasteurian bacteriology) as resulting from the invasion of one's body by external pathogens (colloquially called 'germs' or 'bugs'). Thus we 'catch' flu. It is then the job of the doctor, aided by laboratory tests, backed by science and technology, to destroy this invader, with the aid of miracle drugs, especially antibiotics, and to relieve suffering with pain-killers. Alternatively, other kinds of illness are seen as due to some 'breakdown' in the body's mechanism, the failure of a part such as a hip-joint or the heart; generally in hospital, while the sufferer is unconscious under anaesthetics, this can be mended, or the organ can even be 'replaced'. The patient wakes up better [46].

This outline sketch can be called the 'medical model' of physical illness. Disease is treated as an alien entity. It strikes from outside for no particular reason. It afflicts our 'body' – which is not quite the same as our 'self'. And we trust the doctor to repair the damaged part, rather as we expect garage mechanics to mend our car. Overall, illness has no particular meaning and the doctor is the active agent, the hero even, in its conquest.

Little of this story would have rung true to Tudor or Stuart sufferers, or even to most Victorians. In earlier centuries, illness was standardly seen not as a random assault from outside, but as a deeply significant life-event, integral to the sufferer's whole being, spiritual, moral, physical and life-course, past, present and future. This view partly stemmed from contemporary assumptions about what caused illness. The explanations offered by doctors, reflecting the best classical theories, and the outlooks of lay 'common sense', alike regarded good health as a measure of the orderly workings of the individual constitution, and sickness as a sign of its imbalance. To maintain good health, one needed to ensure proper diet, exercise, evacuations, adequate sleep and the like. It was important to reside in a healthy environment, to regulate one's passions, and be moderate and temperate in habit.

More particularly, the different forces vital for life had to be kept in a sensible balance. The body must not be allowed to become too hot or too cold, too wet or too dry; and this in turn depended upon maintaining the right equilibrium between the key fluids (technically called 'humours') that made the system work – for example, blood or phlegm. Sickness was the outcome when the body balance was disturbed. If the system grew too hot and dry, this came out in fever; if too cool and wet, then it developed a cold. If too little blood were produced, the body lacked nourishment and languished. If excessive blood were generated, for example by eating too much red meat and drinking too much port, one's blood would boil or it would rush to the head; 'hot-blooded' people were liable to apoplexy (a stroke). Thus sickness was largely seen as personal, internal, and brought on by faulty lifestyle. Such 'distempers' (being out of temper) could be treated by restoring the lost equilibrium; hence 'cooling' herbal medicines, blood-lettings or even cold baths would be good for fevers, while plenty of rich food and red meat would cure 'thin blood'. Better still, careful attention to all aspects of 'regimen' or lifestyle, would prevent 'disease' (literally 'dis-ease') in the first place [93].

Thus, from minor discomforts to dangerous fevers and seizures, bouts of sickness were typically seen as hinging on the individual's constitution and personality. This entailed the converse of today's 'doctor dependence': your life was not in his hands but in your own. Such views made good sense at a time when curative medicine was little advanced (as described above in Chapter 1) and the physician's healing power was extremely limited. It also harmonised with an often expressed faith in the 'healing power of nature' (in Latin: *vis medicatrix naturae*), a common-sense recognition of the self-limiting nature of most ailments. One way that people in traditional societies coped with the fact that doctors were not miracle-workers was to treat their health as ultimately a matter of personal responsibility. As will be seen below, this belief had important consequences when it came to deciding what to do on falling sick [3; 96].

If, physiologically and psychologically speaking, keeping well was regarded chiefly as a matter of leading a balanced, regular, moderate life, why did people so often fall sick and die? Several general explanations were widely proposed. For one thing, bad environments or unhealthy occupations were recognized as breeding disease. Ever since the Greeks, it had been common knowledge that overcrowded and airless quarters of towns were hotbeds of epidemics, or that those living in fenny or estuarine areas frequently got 'ague' (malaria). The source lay, it was believed, with poisonous gases (miasmata) given off by the soil and standing water. Only vigorous motion, free currents of air and fast-flowing water would break up and dispel these vapours. Likewise, it was well known that potters got lung diseases and that lead-workers were liable to paralysis: such diseases just came with the job [134]; in those days there was no state regulation of dangerous trades.

Second, it was widely believed that sickness could be the result of spells cast by witches (*maleficium*) or of satanic possession. Belief in witchcraft, magic and sorcery gradually declined after the mid-seventeenth century – precisely how and why remains a subject of fierce historical dispute – and it seems that the attribution of illnesses to evil spirits, and attempts to counter them by magical remedies, slowly became confined to the lower orders, to the countryside, and to oral culture. Nevertheless residues of medical magic – such as passing a child suffering from whooping cough under a donkey – survived into the nineteenth century; and it long remained acceptable amongst certain Christian sects to attribute afflictions to the Devil. In the eighteenth century, John Wesley, the founder of Methodism – and, in his own way, a pioneer of new scientific therapies, like the use of electricity for medical purposes – regarded insanity as routinely caused by diabolical possession [95; 126].

Third, the fallen estate of mankind was widely blamed for the universal empire of sickness, suffering and death. Through Original Sin and the resulting expulsion from Paradise, Adam and Eve had brought disease and death upon the human race as punishments for disobedience; the Bible warned women that, as a result of the Fall, 'in pain thou shalt bring forth children' (Genesis 3:16). Mainstream seventeenth-century Protestantism believed the world was old and decaying fast; and plagues, epidemics, disasters, dearth, famine and wars were widely interpreted as signs that the end was nigh. Disease could thus be a perpetual *memento mori*, a reminder of death, and death itself a release from this vale of tears [41; 64].

Such views could make broad sense of the omnipresence of disease and death. They did not, however, satisfactorily explain the personal dilemma: why did it befall *me*? Today, because most maladies are just passing interludes, we rarely feel the need to endow them with special meanings. In earlier centuries life was precarious, death commonly struck in the very prime of life, and the salvation of the immortal soul was paramount: in such circumstances, each illness episode had to be scrutinised for its deeper portents and meanings. And so, as the musings of contemporary diarists show, sickness was interpreted as packed with moral, spiritual and religious messages. Often it was read as the operation of natural justice. Thus adulterers would contract venereal infections; the idle would be punished with melancholy; and the sins of the parents would be visited upon their children. Even the worldly Pepys sometimes deciphered his ailments as penalties for sexual misdeeds [91; 96].

Above all, sickness was regarded as the finger of Providence. The Lord used illness for a multitude of higher purposes. It could be an affliction to smite the ungodly, like the Old Testament pestilences hurled against the Egyptians. Thus bubonic plague was widely interpreted by the pious as a correction, a reminder of Divine Wrath and a caution to the wicked to mend their ways. But there were positive sides to Providence too. When the Puritan Richard Baxter fell sick and thus escaped involvement in some disagreeable business, he judged the Hand of God had spared him; it was a kind of Divine medical certificate. For the Revd Ralph Josselin in mid-seventeenth century Essex, the fact that the pain of bee stings could be soothed by applying honey was further proof of the benevolence of divine Providence, in supplying ready remedies for doubtless well-deserved afflictions. In any case, physical pain was reckoned to serve as a divine advance warning regarding far more excruciating spiritual torments in Hell. A bee sting alerted Josselin to the incomparably greater dangerous sting of sin [93].

Thus sickness was read as one of the many ways through which God revealed His will to man. Belief that disease had divine meanings did not, however, supplant the idea that it also had natural causes to be handled medically (compare Oliver Cromwell's instruction to his troops to 'trust in God and keep your powder dry'). Few people thought that medicine and the Divine will were at odds, though some Scottish Calvinists later judged it impious to inoculate against smallpox, arguing that if it was God's will that one contracted smallpox, it was wicked to frustrate it. Muslims took few precautions to avoid plague, seeing it as a blessed mark of divine favour. But such religious fatalism was rare in seventeenth-century England. Worries as to how to square Providence with medicine, holiness and healing, seem more common in the nineteenth century, with the emergence of such religious sects as the Christian Scientists.

The medical culture of pre-industrial England thus focused upon the individual, and God's purposes for him, rather than (as today) upon organised, institutionalised medicine. This had important implications for the actions people took in the teeth of illness. For one thing, diaries and letters show that sufferers paid great attention to the causes of sickness and took steps to avoid it. The prudent were meticulous in choosing their diet, in keeping warm (a particular concern of Pepys), and in taking exercise. (Today's diet faddists and joggers could find plenty of predecessors in earlier centuries!). Those who could afford it visited spas like Bath and Buxton, bathing and drinking the waters [47; 112; 127]. Many diarists routinely dosed themselves with tonics, gave themselves purges and emetics, and called in the local barber-surgeon to let blood, as steps in self-administered programmes of health. In the eighteenth and nineteenth centuries, many ways of toughening the constitution and cleansing the system gained a following, including gymnastics, cold-water bathing, vegetarianism and teetotalism. In Victorian times, putting prevention before cure and Nature before the doctors became the hallmark of lay-dominated alternative medicine [10; 56; 97].

Moreover, autobiographical evidence from diaries and letters shows that when people fell sick, they made a point of forming their own diagnosis, rather than leaving it to the doctor. Symptoms were rarely recorded without an accompanying stab at an explanation. When, early in 1663, Samuel Pepys went down with stomach pains and fever, he puzzled deeply as to the cause, deciding it was 'some disorder given the blood: but by what I know not, unless it be by my late great Quantitys of Dantzicke-girkins that I have eaten'. In the face of such danger, it was reassuring to come up with an explanation. It allayed anxiety. But it also helped sufferers to make the next important decision: should they summon professional help or not? Nowadays many people automatically pay a visit to the doctor as soon as they feel sick or below par ('under the weather'). But few folk in early modern society – except of course certain hypochondriacs – routinely sent for the doctor when they felt ill, even badly ill. No one thought that professionals had a monopoly of medical expertise. Nobody regarded it as offensive to their doctor to try self-dosing first, or anticipated incurring his wrath by so doing.

So people pondered their symptoms and attempted their own diagnosis. Very often, they would then administer medical self-help. Well-stocked homes went in for 'kitchen physic', making up bottles of home-brewed purges, vomits, pain-killers, cordials, febrifuges (medicines to reduce fever) and the like. At least by the mid-eighteenth century it was common for families to stock up with shop-bought patent and proprietary medicines such as Dr James' Powders, the Georgian equivalent of aspirin. By the nineteenth century products still familiar today, like Eno's Fruit Salts and Beecham's Pills, were beginning to appear. One could also buy ready-to-use medicine chests. The assistance of friends, family members, 'wise women' or the squire or parson might also be sought. Contemporary letters abound with recipes and treatments recommended in response to news of ailments and accidents. Recipe-books and health-care manuals bulge with home remedies for all kinds of disorders, from corns to cancer [10; 75].

Self-medication is, of course, universal. But the sick a couple of centuries ago were probably far more self-reliant and less doctor-dependent than today. That is not surprising; they had to be. Doctors had no sure-fire bags of tricks. Educated lay-people might reasonably believe – unlike nowadays – that they could talk the same language as the doctor and understand medicine on a par with him. Moreover, in those days, there were no drugs that could be obtained only on prescription. Till well into the nineteenth century, all drugs – even dangerous ones like opium – and poisons too could freely be bought over the counter [10].

But what happened if the sick person decided to call the doctor? Much depended upon social class. Today's general practitioner commands professional authority, partly because he is backed by diagnostic technology, laboratory tests, hospital specialists and consultants, and the general prestige, or mystique, of medical science [111]. Great things are expected of him. That was far from true three centuries ago. Practitioners often came from a lower social rank than their gentry clients; hence they were expected to show due deference. Not least, influential patients clearly expected doctors to fall in with their self-diagnoses and favourite treatments. The eighteenth-century writer, Samuel Johnson – a man who respected doctors, though he was a particularly cantankerous patient – routinely ordered his doctors around. On one occasion, against his physician's advice, he insisted that his surgeon bled him.

Johnson had faith in heroic remedies like blood-letting, believing that 'pop-gun batteries' did no good; a fact which suggests that the fashion for vile-tasting brews crammed with disgusting ingredients may have been to satisfy sick people's need to feel that medicines were really having some effect. At the dawn of the nineteenth century, Dr Thomas Percival, in a pioneering book on medical ethics, advised physicians to fall in with the desires of wealthy paying patients to have their own favourite medicines prescribed – while, of course, denying any such indulgence could be allowed to poor charity patients being treated free in hospitals [57].

In modern doctor-patient relations, the doctor is in the driving seat, so much so that radical critics of the profession, like Ivan Illich, have reiterated George Bernard Shaw's gibe that medicine is 'a conspiracy against the layman' [55]. This would hardly be an apt description for medicine three or four hundred years ago. Back in the sixteenth or seventeenth centuries the profession as a whole commanded little corporate power, and few individual physicians attained great celebrity or wealth. The diaries of eighteenth-century patients show that they often disregarded their physician's advice, and discharged bossy practitioners. They felt no compunction about shopping around for second and third opinions, and made free use of quack and unorthodox remedies as well, following a try-anything philosophy that gave no automatic privilege to regular medicine [93].

In the long run, the collective prestige of doctors would rise, the patient would be more firmly fixed 'under the doctor', and consumers would lose some of their say. These developments will be traced in Chapters 4 and 5. But that rise was slow, and scepticism about the medical profession long continued. Popular proverbs endorsed this distrust ('one doctor makes work for another'), and echoed the Biblical: 'physician, heal thyself'. Physicians were pilloried in popular novels as 'Dr Slop' or 'Dr Smelfungus', and collectively in a famous engraving by William Hogarth as the 'Company of Undertakers'. Many would have agreed with the kind of resignation expressed in 1739 by Elizabeth Montagu:

I have swallowed the weight of an Apothecary in medicine, and what I am better for it, except more patient and less credulous, I know not. I have learnt to bear my infirmities and not to trust to the skills of physicians for curing them. I endeavour to drink deeply of philosophy, and to be wise when I cannot be merry, easy when I cannot be glad, content with what cannot be mended, and patient where there can be no redress. The mighty can do no more, and the wise seldom do as much. [94]

It is perhaps revealing that, up to the end of the seventeenth century, physicians were not routinely present at life's two greatest crises, birth and death. Traditional child-birth was a 'women only' occasion, attended by midwives and 'gossips' (that is, friends and neighbours) but not, except in emergencies, by medical practitioners [9]. Death-beds were similar. The humane doctor would tactfully tell his patients that they were dying, to give them time to put their affairs in order, and, acknowledging that there was no more for him to do, would retire, leaving the last hours to the family and perhaps a clergyman. In the world of traditional medicine – long before intensive care units – sufferers and doctors could co-exist without undue tension, because the limits of medicine's powers were clear to all.

4

Medicine in the market economy of the Georgian age

This survey has been arguing that medicine led a chequered existence in the 'world we have lost'. Although the nation boasted a few great medical scientists – of whom William Harvey, discoverer of the circulation of the blood, and the astute clinician, Thomas Sydenham, are amongst the most eminent – the professional elite had more enemies than friends, and was accused of being monopolistic and self-serving without being able to offer correspondingly successful medical care. Neither the College of Physicians nor the Company of Surgeons did much for medical education or research (the Royal Society, chartered in 1662, was initially somewhat more energetic, staging the first experimental blood transfusions). Attempts by seventeenth-century Puritan reformers and by advocates of the new chemically-based drugs to change the structure of organised medical practice or to establish new theories and therapies met with resistance.

It would be easy to paint a picture of medicine in eighteenth-century England as meandering down the same channel, still unreformed, though still more oligarchic. The Colleges, for example, grew yet more exclusive and nepotistic, mirroring and being sheltered by the Walpolean political system of 'Old Corruption'. Indeed, that is precisely how nineteenth-century reformers, spearheaded by the journal, the *Lancet*, founded in 1823 by the surgeon and democrat, Thomas Wakley, viewed things in their crusades against the medical establishment. Historians have commonly endorsed their reading, seeing the eighteenth century as an era of medical stagnation, destined finally to be swept aside in the 'age of reform' by a new broom that put an end to privilege and patronage, and created the 'career open to talent' [40].

Indeed, there is much to be said for this view. By no criterion did the College of Physicians or the Company of Surgeons improve the standards of English medicine during the 'long eighteenth century'. The College suffered some reverses around 1700, falling out of royal favour, and (after the House of Lords' judgment in the Rose Case, 1704) losing its monopoly right to prescribe medicines in London [20]. Henceforth, the Lords ruled, apothecaries might also prescribe, provided that they charged only for their medicines, not for their advice. (One dubious effect of this otherwise progressive judgment was that it gave apothecaries every incentive to offload increasing quantities of medicines onto their patients.)

Following this defeat, the College of Physicians grew introverted. Over the years, it largely abandoned the attempt to exercise its police powers to prosecute unlicensed practitioners – for this dereliction of duty it was roundly abused by later reformers – turning instead into an exclusive club, reserved for gentlemen physicians. The College successfully frustrated all demands that it open its fellowship to London physicians at large. Its statutes standardly reserved admission into its fellowship – the inner sanctum of power and prestige – to graduates of Oxford and Cambridge and members of the Church of England. Yet, by 1750, many of London's best physicians were Dissenters by religion and had been trained either at Leiden in the Netherlands or at Edinburgh University, which by then boasted perhaps the top medical school in the world [113]. Eminent physicians like the Scot, William Hunter, and the Quakers, John Fothergill and John Coakley Lettsom, ardently resented being forced to remain mere 'licentiates' of the College: non-voting members, or, in other words, second-class citizens. Reformers' campaigns to open up the College met with diehard opposition [17; 129].

The Surgeons' Company likewise made hardly any contribution to medical advance. The formal separation in 1745 of the Surgeons from the Barbers did at least establish that surgery was a craft in itself, a cut above mere hairdressing: but the divorce accidentally spelt a backward step as well, since the new premises occupied by the Surgeons long lacked a dissecting theatre. (One of the *raisons d'être* for the Surgeons' Company lay in its right to conduct public dissections of executed criminals for educational and research purposes – important in an age when anatomical knowledge was seen as vital to every surgeon's training.) [23]

If the London corporation did little for medical education, English universities achieved little more. The output of medical graduates from Oxford and Cambridge during the Georgian era sank far below the levels reached in the previous century. Most medical professors were nonentities, who rarely lectured, and Oxford and Cambridge missed out on one of the key advances in medical education made at Leiden and Edinburgh, the integration of student lectures with clinical instruction in an adjoining hospital [108; 113]. Overall, Georgian England failed to provide medical training adequate to its needs. By the close of the eighteenth century, top London physicians, the cream of provincial physicians, and the leading hospital and army and navy surgeons – an increasingly important branch of the profession – were getting their medical education elsewhere, above all in Edinburgh, which pioneered university education for surgeons, not just for physicians [101; 108; 113].

Last and not least in this diagnosis of Georgian decay, is the fact that medicine remained formally straitjacketed in its traditional, three-tiered, hierarchical structure (in descending order, physicians, surgeons and apothecaries), their relations sometimes soured by rivalry and jealousy. This legal and institutional division of labour had grown archaic and did not conform to the realities of medical need and practice. After all, from 1704 London apothecaries had the right to practise medicine, though not to be paid for it. And in the provinces the great majority of regular medical men, whatever their training or licence, operated neither as physicians, surgeons nor apothecaries, but as all three in one, as general practitioners [6; 69].

The failure of this medical hierarchy to reform meant that Georgian physicians remained sitting targets for satire and censure, being presented as living fossils, clinging to obsolete learning. Yet this is only part of the picture, and not the most important aspect. For overall, medical care grew rapidly in the eighteenth century – in quantity and in quality too – and the standing of many medical practitioners rose alongside. This was the product of various trends [44].

For one thing, a large sector of the population was enjoying unprecedented prosperity. England came to boast a broad and ever-expanding middling class of merchants, tradesmen, shop-keepers, clerks, farmers, skilled craftsmen and the like, with money to spare after the necessities of life had been supplied. Perhaps aping their betters, such families began to spend more upon services, commodities, and consumer items as part of a general commercialisation of living. Amongst the many outlays increasingly recorded in their account books – alongside expenditure on library subscriptions, hairdressers, music lessons and similar services – were payments to medical practitioners. Women whose mothers had relied upon the village midwife now booked the *accoucheur* (male obstetrician or 'man midwife') to deliver their babies [64]; women whose grandmothers had mixed family brews now bought proprietary medicines for their ailments or summoned the surgeon-apothecary. Medicine expanded as part of the widespread growth of the service sector in a thriving, market-oriented consumer economy [5].

At the same time, lay initiatives led to the setting up of new medical institutions. Thinkers propagating the socio-political outlooks of the Enlightenment were keen to promote secular welfare, the *health* alongside the *wealth* of nations. They also set great store by humanitarianism and philanthropy. Certain traditional types of charity, however, notably religious good works and educational foundations, had acquired a dubious reputation for exacerbating sectarian animosities in a society already deeply politically and religiously split. Medical charities, by contrast, many hoped, would prove a balm, healing social wounds not irritating them. Partly for these reasons, the Georgian century witnessed a quite unprecedented spate of private giving for medical good causes – in particular, the founding of hospitals and, somewhat later, of dispensaries. Such institutions were typically meant for the poor (though not for Poor Law paupers), who would receive care without charge, thus, it was hoped, confirming ties of deference, gratitude and paternalism [42].

London benefited earliest from the wave of new foundations. To the metropolis's two ancient hospitals, St Thomas's and St Bartholomew's, a further five were added in quick succession between 1720 and 1750: the Westminster (1720), Guy's (1724), St George's (1733), the London (1740) and the Middlesex (1745) [13; 18;

28; 102]. All these were general hospitals. They set off a chain reaction of similar institutions in the provinces, where, until then, no genuinely 'medical' hospitals had existed at all (earlier 'hospitals' were just alms-houses). The Edinburgh Royal Infirmary was set up in 1729, followed by Winchester and Bristol (1736–7) [35], York (1740), Exeter (1741), Bath (1742), Northampton (1743) and some twenty others. By 1800, all sizable English towns had a hospital [28; 140]. The old corporate towns and cathedral cities got them first, the newer manufacturing centres like Birmingham and Manchester somewhat later.

Augmenting these general foundations, Georgian philanthropy also pumped money into more specialist institutions for the sick, particularly in London, but elsewhere too. Charitable impulses led to St Luke's Hospital being opened in London in 1751, the only big public lunatic asylum in the kingdom apart from Bethlem. Unlike 'Bedlam', which was widely criticised for its supposed barbarity and benightedness, St Luke's was launched to an optimistic and progressive fanfare, its physician, William Battie, asserting that, if treated with humanity, lunacy was as curable as any other disease. By 1800, other great towns, like Manchester, Liverpool and York, had their own public lunatic asylums, philanthropically supported [60; 95].

As well as lunatics, sufferers from venereal disease also became objects for charity, perhaps indicating a waning of the traditional religious judgment that such diseases were retribution for vice, and its replacement by the enlightened view that humanity demanded relief of suffering. London's 'Lock Hospital' for venereal cases opened in 1746. It was paralleled by another new charitable foundation, the Magdalen Hospital for Penitent Prostitutes (1759). That was less a medical hospital than a refuge, in which prostitutes who wished to mend their ways could stay, learn a trade, and prepare for a new life. Another important type of new voluntary hospital was the lying-in hospital. In London, the earliest of these maternity hospitals were the British (1749), the City (1750), the General (1752) and the Westminster (1765). Maternity hospitals met several major needs. Not least, they guaranteed a few days' bed-rest to poor women living in overcrowded tenements and overwhelmed by the incessant demands of large families. Also, because some did not insist that the mother-to-be should be married, they enabled unmarried mothers – commonly servant girls – to deliver their illegitimate offspring with no questions asked. Many of these babies then ended up at the Foundling Hospital, opened in 1741 as London's first major orphanage. Unwanted infants could be deposited there anonymously; they were then nursed, educated and taught a trade [70; 85].

Lying-in hospitals served a further function. From the start they were centres of tuition and practice for trainee midwives and for the newer male *accoucheurs* (man-midwives or obstetricians). All these desirable functions were offset by one grave drawback. In pre-bacteriology days, before sepsis was understood and the need for scrupulous cleanliness recognised, maternity hospitals readily became deathtraps. Mother and baby mortality was higher in these hospitals than with home deliveries [128].

One further important mode of medical charity developed from the 1770s: the dispensary movement. Hospitals aimed to provide treatment, nourishing food and bed-rest, and by 1800, London's hospitals were alone handling between 20,000 and 30,000 patients a year. But hospitals restricted themselves to minor complaints that would respond to treatment, excluded infectious fever victims (it would have been irresponsible to risk having epidemics raging uncontrollably through the infirmary), and in any case, could treat only a fraction of the sick. Hence it became important to augment hospital facilities. One device was the fever hospital, designed only for infectious cases. London's fever hospital (diplomatically known as the House of Recovery) was opened in 1801. If it could do little for typhus, dysentery or diphtheria cases, it could at least help halt the spread of such infections by isolating their victims. But the key device supplementing the hospital was the dispensary. The first London dispensary was set up in 1773. By 1800, sixteen dispensaries existed in London, treating up to 50,000 cases a year; many were founded in the provinces besides. Dispensaries mainly provided outpatient services, supplying advice and free medicine to the sick poor for whom there was no room in hospitals or whose complaints were unsuitable for hospitalisation. Equally important, the dispensary system involved domiciliary visits by eminent physicians into the dwellings of the poor. This first-hand experience of how the other half lived fired the reforming zeal of progressive doctors, leading to agitation for improved housing, better sanitation and health education for the people [11; 68].

These initiatives transformed the English medical landscape. True, the voluntary hospital movement did not amount to the comprehensive, state-funded medical system that certain seventeenth-century Puritans had envisaged (that had to wait until 1948). Neither did it spark any major breakthroughs in medical science or therapeutic capacity: it is one thing to provide a VD hospital or a lunatic asylum, and another to cure the victims of such disorders. Such foundations did, however, signal a new recognition on the part of influential elites that the people's health mattered. Piety and humanity demanded compassion for the sick; economics and utility taught that neglecting disease ran counter to enlightened self-interest: for diseases readily spread from the poor to the better off, and sick and incapacitated labourers made inefficient employees. In the light of these moral considerations, it is not surprising that initiatives for institutional advances generally sprang from laymen, not doctors. Thomas Guy, whose benefaction set up Guy's Hospital, was a London printer; Thomas Coram, inspirer of the Foundling Hospital, was an old sea-dog, distressed to see babies abandoned on the streets of the capital [70]; Alured Clarke, who drew up the blueprints for many provincial voluntary hospitals, was a clergyman. Subscriptions for such foundations generally came from nobles and gentlemen, rich merchants, clergy and civic worthies: and as generous donations carried votes on governing boards, the management of these hospitals and charities largely remained in the hands of the laity, with physicians taking a back seat.

Of course, the hospital movement greatly benefited the medical profession as well. Every hospital had one or more honorary appointments for physicians and surgeons. They would give their services free (or for a nominal honorarium) as an act of public generosity. The honour and publicity accruing from hospital appointments proved valuable career 'leg-ups' for ambitious practitioners, who could expect, through the hospital, to hobnob with the governors and gentry, and thereby gain powerful patrons and wealthy private patients. Hospital appointments, especially in London, could prove more directly lucrative as well: hospital staff, especially surgeons, took apprentices who would walk the wards, and learn the craft while acting as the surgeon's assistant. It was the ideal apprenticeship, and the surgeon could command good fees. Moreover, especially after about 1750, London hospital doctors began to deliver lecture courses on hospital premises on such subjects as anatomy, pharmacy, surgery and practical medicine. Popular courses drew scores of students; the fees they paid would entitle them not just to attend lectures but to have access to the hospital wards. Thus the habit grew up of 'walking the wards': generally, the students were in tow to the physician or surgeon as he did his rounds, explaining cases as he went from patient to patient: sometimes they inspected on their own [42; 50].

Thus hospital expansion gave rise to teaching in the hospitals, accompanied by the growing practice of dissection [35; 104]. Even if this was not as formal or systematic as the medical education provided, from the early Victorian era, by 'teaching hospitals' proper (for instance, University College or King's College Hospital), it at least represented a great educational leap forward, by bringing together theoretical and practical instruction. If English universities did nothing in the eighteenth century for improving medical education, voluntary hospitals made up for some of their defects [9; 81; 101].

The hospital movement thus provided benefits for the medical profession. It began as a lay initiative. It showed that the polite and the propertied recognised that if capitalism was to enjoy security it must wear a human face; they saw that the wealth of nations depended upon the productive toil of the respectable labouring classes; common sense taught it was prudent to keep such people fit for work. Gradually, however, physicians and especially surgeons began to take the initiative in the day-to-day running of hospitals. In the nineteenth century, the special nature of the hospital, with its large numbers of poor patients suffering from similar conditions, encouraged major new initiatives in medical theory and practice [42].

These medical initiatives were also a response to the fact that in a free-market, industrialising society which was deploying more powerful and dangerous machinery and highly toxic chemicals, working people were increasingly being stricken by industrial accidents and occupational diseases. A few employers, notably the potter Josiah Wedgwood, set up private sickness insurance schemes, through which the workforce, in return for compulsory deductions from their wages, received entitlements to medical treatment and sick pay. But masters and employers of domestic servants more commonly chose to make contributions to hospital charities, which would qualify them for admittance tickets for their employees.

Specialised medical charities offer further evidence of an awareness of the hazards of industrialization. The Royal Humane Society, founded in 1773, aimed to teach techniques of artificial resuscitation to save those rescued from drowning. With shipping, ports, rivers and canals playing a key role in economic expansion, many fell victim to the hazards of water (children were not generally taught to swim) – and it was also said that the proverbially suicidal English made a habit of throwing themselves off bridges in despair. Other bodies were set up to provide free surgical appliances to those in heavy manual labour whose working-life was threatened by hernias and ruptures. All such institutions continued to function and expand throughout the nineteenth century, indeed up to the founding of the National Health Service [134].

There was thus recognition of the benefits offered by expanding medical provision, both private and public. Doctors in their turn eagerly cashed in upon the new opportunities; the eighteenth century saw the practice of medicine flourishing as never before. At the pinnacle of the profession, the Georgian medical elite grew more fashionable, more prestigious, more well-to-do than its Stuart equivalent. This rise had little to do with any new and dramatically effective medical skills. It was more a matter of top physicians acquiring a veneer of culture and urbanity, and thus turning themselves into the kind of well-bred men High Society, and in particular society ladies, felt they could trust and admit to their circles. Such physicians as William Hunter (obstetrician to fashionable society), John Coakley Lettsom, William Heberden and Matthew Baillie won faithful clienteles, widespread commendation and social approbation through their clinical acumen and through a courteous good breeding that avoided old-fashioned pedantry and uncouthness [9]. Other physicians made their mark by excelling as cultural leaders or literary lions. Both Richard Mead and Sir Hans Sloane dabbled in science and built up fabulous collections of antiquities, books and *objets d'art* (bequeathed to the nation, Sloane's collection became the nucleus of the British Museum). The surgeon William Cheselden was a friend of Alexander Pope and designed a bridge over the Thames at Putney. Others won *entrée* as men of letters: Samuel Garth, Richard Blackmore, Mark Akenside and Erasmus Darwin were probably equally famous as poets and as physicians; Tobias Smollett and Oliver Goldsmith were doctors whose literary careers outstripped their medical.

For those at the top of the tree, incomes soared. William Cheselden could reputedly charge £500 for a lithotomy operation (removing a bladder stone). That was a splendid 'piece' rate, since his forte lay in extracting stones in under five minutes: before anaesthetics, brevity was the soul of surgery. (£500 was the annual income of many a country squire.) Lettsom, Mead, Hunter and Baillie all probably topped £10,000 a year, an income unknown in earlier centuries and equivalent to the annual income of a minor lord [9].

But better times spread throughout the profession. Recent research has shown that the fees small-town apothecaries and country surgeons could command steadily rose during the eighteenth century [69; 47]. Business also became brisker. A provincial physician like Erasmus Darwin, based first in Lichfield and then in Derby, netted over £1000 a year in the latter part of the century; energetic country general practitioners could earn £500, while a few provincial apothecaries, like William Broderip of Bristol, had incomes running into thousands. Whereas their predecessors had gone on horseback, such men gadded around in carriages and bought themselves country seats. Doubtless they toiled hard for their rewards (Erasmus Darwin believed he travelled 10,000 miles a year on calls); and no doubt only a few did so well, though all the signs point to a substantial upward trend of medical incomes in a century which was, before the 1780s, inflation-free. Overall, Georgian affluence, together with the secular temper of an Enlightenment age in which the claims of the body began to take precedence over those of the soul, spelt good times for doctors [48; 69].

Doctors were helped, furthermore, by the growth of advantageous sidelines. As already noted, hospital posts became available, offering prestige and admission into the higher circles of town life, and the promise of future profit. Other country practitioners topped up their income by engaging in 'contract' Poor Law practice. The developing medical speciality of man-midwifery provided further opportunities. A specialist London man-midwife could charge fees running into hundreds of guineas to deliver titled ladies who found it more modish and perhaps safer to have a well-trained, genteel male practitioner rather than the conventional midwife [64]. Outside London, childbirth was increasingly in the hands of surgeon-apothecaries. They shrewdly perceived that the doctor who successfully delivered a baby won lasting gratitude and, most probably, the mother and child as patients for life. Obstetrics paved the way for the triumph of the family doctor in the nineteenth century [117].

Another well-paying new sideline could be smallpox inoculation. Inoculation (intentionally infecting healthy people with a mild dose of smallpox, to provide future immunity against what often proved a fatal, or, at least, a dangerous and disfiguring disease) had been introduced into England in the 1720s by Lady Mary Wortley Montagu (a lay person, not a doctor), who had seen it deployed as a peasant practice in Turkey. The English medical profession proved rather receptive – more than the French – and the practice was given good publicity by the willingness of the royal family to have their children inoculated. From mid-century, inoculation was widely practised (it worked best in small communities, where mass inoculation was feasible). Often it was performed by everyday surgeons, who might charge a guinea a jab. But certain practitioners set themselves up as specialist inoculators. The most successful were the Sutton family. In twenty years Thomas Sutton and his sons, common provincial surgeons, claimed to have performed a staggering 300,000 inoculations, bringing an annual income of several thousand pounds. Even luckier was Thomas Dimsdale. A country physician who had made inoculation his forte, he was invited in 1768 to St Petersburg by Catherine the Great to inoculate her and her son. His reward was £10,000, plus £2000 expenses and an annuity of £500 [76; 104].

In fact, various new routes to fame and fortune were opening for the medics. Some, like John Pringle, chose to make a name for themselves in army or navy medicine: in an epoch of constant warfare and imperial expansion, military medicine offered splendid career prospects for enterprising young doctors with nerves of steel. Pringle rose to become President of the Royal Society [61; 67]. Others began to specialise. As earlier described, traditional medical theory, following Greek views, had seen sickness as a symptomatic disorder of the whole system (the 'constitution') rather than as specific to a particular organ; committed to holism, it tended to denigrate as a quack the practitioner who professed to treat a single condition or organ in isolation – such might be the fate even of eye-doctors who operated for cataract. But circumstances gradually modified this state of affairs. In particular, Edinburgh University was turning out increasing numbers of highly skilled graduates, trained equally in physic and surgery, whose prospects of becoming a fashionable London bedside physician were thwarted by the restrictive practices of the College of Physicians. In the late eighteenth-century and beyond, many such Scottish graduates turned to specialisation as their way up the career ladder. Some, as already mentioned, became man-midwives. Eye, nose, throat specialists followed. Certain practitioners began to specialise in women's and children's disorders [78].

Others turned their energies to medical instruction. From early Georgian times, a handful of practitioners were giving lecturecourses for students in London and, by the close of the century, teaching was standardly being offered in the hospitals. Several enterprising practitioners established their own private anatomy schools in the metropolis, the most famous being set up by the Scot, William Hunter, in Great Windmill Street, Piccadilly, in 1765. Proprietors of anatomy schools gave extensive medical instruction to all who could pay the fee of a few guineas – Hunter's course ran to 112 two-hour sessions. Above all, they catered for the practical side of the art, by providing plenty of demonstrations and pathological specimens preserved in bottles and showcases; and, a key innovation, they gave students first-hand anatomical experience by providing corpses for dissection. For this, entrepreneurs like Hunter had to enter into shady and illegal dealings with London's underworld of body snatchers ('resurrection men'). Private anatomy schools offered the best medical education in London until they were superseded by the teaching hospitals from the 1830s [9; 22; 105].

A further fertile field of medical specialisation affording new career openings was the management of lunacy. Before 1700, the insane were rarely locked up in madhouses. England's only public madhouse, Bethlem Hospital, housed little more than about a hundred lunatics. As noted above, a number of public asylums were set up during the eighteenth century, under philanthropic initiatives. But the main growth came in the private sector. There the 'trade in lunacy' emerged, based upon the private madhouse. Enterprising doctors and keepers would set up premises for confining the insane, charging stiff fees to the friends and family of affluent patients, and lower fees to parish lunatics. In some, the insane were merely kept in safe custody; in the more ambitious asylums, early versions of psychiatric therapy were also given. Private madhouses were profitable business ventures in the free-market economy. They remained utterly unregulated by law until 1774, and thereafter, though licensed, were still subject to little effective supervision. The worst were abuse-riddled; patients were mistreated, and sane people were sometimes confined in them just to keep them out of the way [87; 95].

Some of these private asylums, however, were reputable institutions run by high-minded doctors anxious to specialise in insanity and develop psychiatric expertise. A typical Edinburgh medical graduate, Dr Thomas Arnold set up an asylum in Leicester and published a pioneering two-volume psychiatric textbook. He won the applause of Samuel Johnson's friend and biographer, James Boswell, who had a disturbed brother who had to be locked up, and who was no stranger to depression himself. More spectacular, however, was the success of the Revd Dr Francis Willis, a Church of England clergyman who had turned to medicine and set up his own high-class private asylum at Gretford in Lincolnshire. When George III became delirious in 1788 and his general physicians failed to quieten him, Willis was called in. His bluntness with the King (he put him in a straitjacket) and his unorthodox treatments, which included 'fixing' his patients with his 'eye', a kind of mesmerism, caused disquiet, but George recovered (if only temporarily), Willis took the credit, and was voted a pension of £1000 a year by Parliament.

Insanity was to remain an auspicious field for the enterprising doctor. Unlike in Catholic countries where religious healing orders bore the brunt of care, in England the field was left free for individual madhouse proprietors, who did not even need to be medically qualified. Not until 1845 was it compulsory for local authorities to build asylums, to be charged to the rates. Even after then, most mad people from respectable families remained confined in the seclusion of private asylums. Thus insanity proved yet another condition which doctors steadily made their patch during the eighteenth and nineteenth centuries, a further opportunity for medical practitioners to thrive in England's flourishing and largely *laissez-faire* society [60; 87].

It would be easy to jump to the conclusion that regular medicine grew during the Georgian and early Victorian eras at the expense of lay and unorthodox practice. Midwives certainly felt they were being elbowed out by the ambitious new *accoucheurs*; the 'wise woman' receded into the shadows; and the Victorian antiquarians who patiently collected medical folk-lore believed they were witnessing a dying tradition.

Yet many fields of irregular medicine were actually growing in tandem with the expansion of regular physic, surgery and the apothecaries' trade. In other words, the total national appetite for medicine was rising fast, and the public which, in a free market, ultimately voted with its wallet, was eager to sample whatever therapies, drugs and systems of treatment were on offer. One sort of medicine created business for another. After all, regular medicine had no corner on effectiveness: and although plague had mercifully quit England after 1666, the eighteenth and nineteenth centuries proved to be times when epidemic infections had lost none of their power to kill, while certain 'new' diseases, like rickets, consumption (tuberculosis) and typhus, associated with wretched urban living conditions, grew more common. Whereas medical practice remained quite strictly regulated in the German states and France [103; 112], with regard to medicine, English law and government largely followed the free market maxim of *caveat emptor* ('let the buyer beware'). Irregulars, quacks and patent-medicine vendors capitalised on the opportunities a medicine-hungry market offered. With good reason, the eighteenth century has been called 'the golden age of quackery'.

To speak of quackery is not automatically to impeach the motives of 'empirics' (that is, unqualified practitioners) and nostrum-mongers, nor to pass judgment on their cures as necessarily ineffective. Many of the most famous (or infamous) Georgian quacks, for instance, James Graham, advocate of mud-bathing, vegetarianism and sexual rejuvenation, were fanatics, not cynical exploiters but fervent believers in their own powers and pills. Proprietary remedies were often remarkably similar to those physicians prescribed, sharing the same active ingredients such as opium (used as a pain-killer) and antimony (which induced sweating to reduce fever). In this case, it could make good economic sense for the sick to prefer ready-made remedies simply because they were cheaper. In fact, the best way to approach quackery is to view it as the most entrepreneurial sector of medicine. Few 'empirical' practitioners were regularly trained, unorthodox methods were to the fore, including the use of electric shock therapy, and they drummed up custom by advertising and spectacular publicity, rather than by cultivating a settled general practice by patronage or word-of-mouth recommendation. Quacks made their profits out of selling commodities, above all, nostrums, rather than from receiving fees for advice, expertise and bedside attendance [10; 97].

The traditional Italian-style charlatan, gaudily dressed and aided by a joke-telling stooge and a monkey, setting up his stage on the street corner, drawing a crowd and then drawing some teeth, giving out a few free bottles of julep and selling a few dozen more, and then riding out of town fast, was by no means extinct in Georgian England. Such figures could still cut a dash and make a fortune; even in the late nineteenth century 'Sequah', an 'American' mountebank, created a national sensation by performing 'Red Indian' rituals and vending socalled Indian remedies [115].

Most mountebanks, however, were probably small-timers, like the man who had a circuit in mid-eighteenth century rural Sussex (where regular doctors were few and far between); the local diarist, Thomas Turner, chauvinistically noted that *he* had seen through the fellow, though his wife was taken in. Some, however, made big money. Joanna Stephens hawked a remedy that promised to dissolve painful bladder stones without perilous surgery. Eventually Parliament raised a £5000 subscription to buy the recipe from her. Joshua Ward made a fortune out of his 'pill and drop' nostrum, effective for all diseases. Ward struck it lucky by manipulating George II's dislocated thumb back into place. In the eighteenth century, Samuel Solomon, William Brodum and numerous others, and in the nineteenth, James Morison, Thomas Holloway and Thomas Beecham, all got rich out of proprietary medicines. One clever ploy was to offer to meet needs that regular medicine failed to supply. Thus patent medicines promised to cure otherwise fatal diseases such as TB, or to restore lost youth and vigour, or to treat conditions like sexually transmitted diseases about which patients might be embarrassed to consult their regular physicians. For instance, Solomon's 'Balm of Gilead' claimed to cure the alleged ill-effects of masturbation, while 'Hooper's Female Pills' were a barely disguised abortifacient.

Leading entrepreneurs of the Industrial Revolution, like Josiah Wedgwood, owed their success in part to exploiting consumer psychology and dextrously manipulating publicity and advertising. Similar arts were perfected by the leading lights of irregular medicine. Large promises, attractive packaging, seductive names, free gifts, special offers, money-back-if-not-satisfied guarantees and other razzmatazz, were the common coin of these pioneers of the pharmaceutical industry. Nostrum-mongers above all went in for saturation advertising – in the streets, and then endlessly in the newspapers, London and provincial, that became an all-present feature of Georgian life. Newspaper agents acted as agents for distributing medications, so that country readers might find access to 'mail order' patent medicines easier than to regular doctors.

In these ways, eighteenth- and nineteenth-century medical opportunists cashed in on the self-diagnosing, self-help medical traditions deeply ingrained amongst the laity, while pandering to new 'consumerist' desires for miracle cures and something new. Habits were built up of self-dosing with 'over-the-counter' medicines. Alongside addicts like the poet, Samuel Coleridge and the writer, Thomas De Quincey, the Victorian lower classes and their children swallowed gallons of laudanum, an opium mixture that eased pain and stupefied infants. The 'stop smoking fast' promises of today's small-ads columns and the millions of bottles of useless cough syrups taken even now, are the legacy of the transformation of medicine into a commodity in the first 'consumer revolution'.

The development of a market-oriented, mass-sales medicine did not necessarily amount to alternative medicine, if by that we mean forms of practice radically at odds with orthodoxy (for instance,

herbalism or homœopathy), advanced by opponents of the domi-
nant medical elite [56; 97]. Indeed, the top 'quacks' of Georgian
England are more noteworthy for their desire to be accepted in
smart society than for being anti-establishment champions of the
health of the people. Such quacks as Joshua Ward hobnobbed in
High Society and with top doctors. A little string-pulling ensured
that Ward's 'pill and drop' became standard navy issue. For their
part, too, regular doctors were not averse to profiting from
nostrum-mongering. Dr James' Fever Powders were the patent of
a *bona fide* Oxford MD, respectable medical author, and friend of
Samuel Johnson.

By the nineteenth century, things were changing somewhat.
Both religious dissenters and political radicals were rejecting the
values of the titled, opulent and the fashionable. Instead, sturdy
individualism, liberty, purity and self-help came to represent the
ideals of self-improvement embraced by the artisans and labouring
men of the industrial Midlands and North. Such radicals commonly wanted to have little to do with orthodox medicine or with
the shop-bought medicines they identified with Mammon. Instead
they embraced a new medical sectarianism that went hand-in-hand
with religious nonconformity and political radicalism. For some,
mainly the bourgeoisie, homœopathy had an appeal. Its hostility to
medical profiteering and its stress on the need for absolutely pure
drugs struck chords with clean-living types. More widespread in
appeal were various kinds of 'medical botany' (herbalism), including the Thomsonian or Coffinite movements, introduced from
America at the beginning of the Victorian era. Herbal remedies,
taken straight from nature and often compounded by the sufferers
themselves, ruled out professional exploitation and adulteration,
and were thus the very essence of self-help. Jesse Boot, the founder
of Boots Pure Drug Company, had his roots in medical botany,
setting up as a manufacturer of pharmaceuticals because he was
dissatisfied with the impurities of the drugs then available [10; 16;
56].

This chapter has explored how perceptions of health needs
changed, and were met, in an expanding capitalist society under-
going rapid industrial change. Affluence and secularisation led to
greater resources being diverted into health care, and medicine
increasingly took the form of a commodity in the early years of

industrialisation. Like so many other occupations, medicine prof-
ited in these sunshine years, increasing in numbers and creating
new niches for itself. Medicine became a more lucrative profession,
and doctors were to occupy more prestigious places in society; in
certain manufacturing towns, like Manchester, they rose to
become civic luminaries [90]. Certain historians have argued that
this growing medical presence amounted to 'medicalisation', medicine claiming authority over widening sectors of life [55]. But to
regard English developments in these terms obscures more than it
clarifies – at least before quite late in the nineteenth century. For
despite individual prosperity, regular medicine continued to exercise little collective public power, and enjoyed hardly any state
backing. Almost no British doctors held state employment before
Queen Victoria came to the throne in 1837 [92]. Doctors were still
largely beholden to their clients, and the public was showing itself
notoriously restive and fickle in its choice of what kinds of
medicine to prefer [59].

5

The medical profession and the state in the nineteenth century

In 1823 the surgeon and democrat Thomas Wakley founded a radical medical journal, the *Lancet*. Son of a Devonshire farmer, Wakley was an uncompromising, belligerent radical who fought in boxing booths in his youth, once walked from Devon to London, and adopted the style of a bruiser in his editorials, taking on the medical establishment. Indeed, early readers of the *Lancet* might be pardoned if they got the impression that English medicine was rotten to the core. Wakley shot deadly blasts at all the medical corporations, accusing them of neglecting their duties even as they abused their powers. London hospitals were nests of nepotism, one consequence of which was that the sick suffered neglect, mistreatment and hamfisted surgery. Privileged institutions purporting to protect the public in fact damaged its health. No wonder, argued the *Lancet*, people patronised the equally awful sharks and swindlers whose careers as quacks ought to have been terminated by decisive Collegiate action. In the midst of this ocean of corruption, only the honest surgeon-apothecary, that is, the emergent general practitioner, upheld the standards of true medicine; and for his pains, he could hardly make a decent living [98; 121].

We must take Wakley's whingeings with a pinch of salt. A man of passion and prejudice, he habitually dipped his pen in bile. The early nineteenth century did see dissatisfaction mounting, but that stemmed perhaps less from the feeling that the profession had reached rock bottom, than from a determination to secure better times ahead. Medicine began to grow militant.

Wakley certainly got one element of his diagnosis spot on, however. He grasped how the different branches of medicine were at loggerheads with each other (he was not averse to exploiting their divisions for tactical advantage). Central to his account of medicine's toils and troubles was the view that it would never enjoy its proper place and authority in society, which he believed should be considerable, while it remained fragmented into the antagonistic and obsolescent branches of physic, surgery and pharmacy, each headed by a self-perpetuating cabal that failed to represent the true interests of the bulk of its practitioners. Until the profession was reorganised, the sick could not be protected, fraudulent practitioners silenced, or the public served.

A farsighted parliamentary statesman could possibly have seized the nettle in 1800, 1820 or 1840, and restructured the profession from top to toe. He would have received few thanks for his pains, and no politician reckoned it was his business – let alone his benefit – to clean out the profession's Augean stables on its behalf. Early in the nineteenth century, parliamentary bills designed to alter the regulation of medicine were often introduced but rarely passed; most that did get through were the work of MPs favourable to the wishes of the College of Physicians. Such was the Apothecaries Act of 1815.

This Act was the equivocal outcome of years of reformist agitation by provincial general practitioners, who declared their livelihoods were being undercut by unfair competition from 'mere' druggists, and complained their interests were not protected by any of the London corporations. The Act itself specified that, in future, the normal qualification for practice as an apothecary should be possession of a licence issued by the Society of Apothecaries (the LSA), which involved an apprenticeship, taking stipulated courses, some hospital experience, and passing examinations. This represented a minor victory for general practitioners, since it established a distinct legal boundary separating the qualified apothecary from lowlier medical tradesmen treading on their tails, such as retail druggists [10; 51].

But on the wider issues, it spelt a major jolt to the hopes of the general practitioner, since nothing was done to outlaw or regulate unqualified druggists – or any other quacks and empirics – or to give general practitioners, who constituted perhaps 90 per cent of all medical regulars, a governing body of their own [51; 52].

The aftermath of the 1815 Apothecaries Act was recrimination rather than reconciliation. The divisions within the profession remained. Securely in the saddle, London physicians and surgeons were wilfully deaf to the argument that in a rapidly transforming nation, whose population almost doubled from 6 million in 1760 to 11.3 million in 1820, new problems, new expectations and new standards of medical education and skill required the restructuring of the profession. The Corporations were happy to chug along as before. Further waves of reformist agitation arose in the 1820s and 1830s, including a campaign by rank-and-file surgeons against the self-perpetuating narrow oligarchy running the College of Surgeons. Ordinary members of the College (MRCSs) had no vote in choosing its Council, which co-opted itself.

In the 1830s, in an atmosphere dominated by Parliamentary Reform and by the advent of the cholera pandemic of 1831–32 (which only confirmed the ineffectiveness of medicine) [31; 77; 88], the British Medical Association was founded as a ginger group for GPs aiming to open up the medical corporations on a democratic basis to all their members. But still the medical old guard carried sufficient clout in government circles to maintain the status quo [89; 130].

The reconstitution of the medical profession was not achieved until the 1850s. Again the internal pressure came from below. By the mid-nineteenth century, the medical profession was, numerically speaking, utterly dominated by non-metropolitan general practitioners. There may formerly have been some sense in keeping them as a subordinate element, back in the days when the typical country surgeon was an old sawbones and the apothecary kept shop, and neither knew more medicine than an apprenticeship had taught them. But that situation was long past. Many country practitioners now had a top-class medical degree, from Edinburgh, Glasgow, or, in a growing trickle, from the newly-founded London University. Those lacking a degree were generally now both Licentiates of the Society of Apothecaries (LSA) and Members of the Royal College of Surgeons (MRCS). A large number now held responsible public office, as Poor Law doctors, as physicians to public lunatic asylums, or as surgeons to public hospitals. The disfranchisement of such men from their own professional bodies was becoming a scandal apparent both to alert leaders of the profession and to politicians.

For the fear was that unless regular medicine had reform imposed upon it by Parliament – it showed no sign of truly reforming itself – it would forfeit public confidence and lose ground to the other kinds of medicine – commercial medicine such as druggists offered, fringe medicine and the medical sects, eventually suffering the fate of the medical regulars in the USA where, without legislative protection, orthodox medicine seemed to be losing to the sects in the battle for public favour [122].

Alongside several less important subsequent pieces of legislation, the Medical Act of 1858 proved an ingenious compromise, placating the reformers, protecting the profession, and ensuring that in the resultant readjustment of territorial boundaries, no branch of the regular profession came out as losers. To satisfy the Colleges of Physicians and of Surgeons, the tripartite division of English medicine was not abolished: the Colleges themselves survived unscathed. To satisfy general practitioners, however, these distinctions became for practical purposes meaningless. In future one single public register for all legally recognised practitioners would be published, under the official authorisation of a General Medical Council (GMC). All names would appear equally on it, from the plushest Harley Street consultant down to the humblest village LSA. The significance of the Register lay, of course, in those it excluded. For all ranks of regular practitioners now appeared together, cheek-by-jowl, as 'insiders', lined up against all the 'outsiders' – the unqualified homœopaths, medical botanists, quacks, bone-setters, itinerants and the like, who were automatically constituted, by exclusion, into the 'fringe'. Parliament had achieved what the doctors could never; it had, symbolically at least, united the much-divided medical profession, by defining them over and against a common Other, not to say enemy [89; 130].

Moreover, the Medical Act had teeth, though not a very powerful bite. Thenceforth it became a legal offence for those not on the Medical Register to represent themselves as medical practitioners (an offence akin to false pretences). To the chagrin of GPs however, the practice of healing by non-registered doctors was in no way made illegal. Parliament knew that any such ban would have been exceedingly unpopular with the public and anyway utterly impossible to enforce. Practitioners not on the register, however, were disqualified from holding public medical office.

Since large numbers of doctors were gaining full or part-time paid public employment as Medical Officers of Health, Poor Law infirmary doctors, forensic experts in the courts, asylum superintendents and so forth, this was a privilege worth having.

This public unification of the divided profession found institutional expression. The Colleges of Physicians and Surgeons remained, as did the Society of Apothecaries; but they were little more than ghosts of past glories. Henceforth two bodies would carry greater weight within the modernised profession. On the one hand, the British Medical Association (BMA) grew out of its rebellious youth as the GPs ginger group, and settled down to become the sober, conservative voice of the profession, aided by its mouthpiece, the *British Medical Journal*. On the other, the General Medical Council (GMC) became the parliamentarily sanctioned official watchdog of medicine (though its members mainly came from within the profession). Its fundamental function was guardianship of the Register. The GMC would add names to the Register. More crucially, it would be the body that struck names off, for such offences as gross professional misconduct (expulsion rarely happened). Through the GMC, the state gave its blessing to medicine's claims to be an autonomous, self-governing ethical profession.

The constitutional reorganisation of the 1850s has proved durable; this was partly because it mainly registered changes the profession had already undergone. For, long before the 1858 Act ended the paper wars between physicians, surgeons and apothecaries, new professional regroupings had taken shape. London's elite physicians and surgeons had ceased to require the cumbersome armour that Collegiate privileges provided. They were successfully establishing themselves in new, secure and well-upholstered positions of eminence and authority. They had increasingly associated themselves with hospital medicine: prestigious not because of its patients, but because of the opportunities it provided for prominence in teaching, for gathering pupils, for making a scientific name, for exercising patronage, and for winning public recognition. The distinction of a practice in Harley Street, combined with a consultancy at a leading London hospital, with patients recommended by one's former pupils for whom one had found good practices in choice areas: these features ensured that medicine continued extremely hierarchical even after the old hierarchy was in effect undermined [89; 100].

For the GP in Rochdale or Rotherham, however, the professional recognition – the semi-closed shop – offered by the mid-Victorian legislation amounted to little. He was a member of an ancient, learned, liberal profession and had probably invested in his training far more time, energy and expense than his father or grandfather. But his prospects depended almost wholly upon the market forces of supply and demand. Things worked out nicely for some. A senior practitioner in a county town like Winchester, serving as honorary physician to the local voluntary hospital, might be fortunate both in income and in status. But such were in a minority. For many GPs winds blew chill in Victorian times. Much of the problem lay in the fact that the profession was growing overstocked. There were all too few genteel career openings for the Victorian middle classes who didn't want to soil their hands with trade. Medicine fitted the credentials for a liberal profession – but it fitted them all too well. By mid-century, Edinburgh, Glasgow, Oxbridge and London University were, between them, turning out hundreds of medical graduates a year. This number increased still further with the founding of provincial university medical schools later in the century. Without plenty of pull and capital to buy themselves into an established practice, too many graduates were faced by the prospect of lean years of desultory practice in a provincial town, waiting for senior rivals to die off, often involving exploitation as a junior partner, in which the senior would treat his underling as a dogsbody while pocketing most of the fees. Dr Arthur Conan Doyle, a young GP in Southsea, took to writing detective stories because he had so few patients.

Reform-minded general practitioners had hoped that raising the admission requirements for the profession, forming a register and penalising unregistered practice would do the trick. But it did not. The only way GPs' financial prospects could be guaranteed to rise would have lain in curbing entry into the medical schools, and pruning the graduate lists. But such 'restrictive practices' would have smacked too much of old Collegiate oligarchy or new trade unionism.

One need not shed too many tears over the living standards of Victorian GPs. Nevertheless, it is not clear that most fared better than their forebears, the Georgian surgeon-apothecaries. To that extent, to speak of the rise of the GP, though true in one respect, hides an irony: to many it seemed more like a decline. Few secured a competent living (and all that that entailed, including the ability to marry respectably and start a family) before they were approaching forty. Most remained appallingly overworked, on call at all hours, fifty-two weeks a year. They had to be endlessly civil to snobbish affluent patients, willing to bear with slow payers and inured to bad debts. They also had to uphold raised professional standards. Most ended up, willy-nilly, treating scores of the sick poor who never paid at all. And rivals were always snapping at their heels [69].

Particularly in the early stages of a career, doctors often had to engage in practice that was arduous, distasteful and barely remunerative. Many young GPs became Poor Law doctors or workhouse medical officers, under the terms of the New Poor Law (1834): agreeing to meet the medical needs of a 'union' of parishes at least guaranteed an income of a couple of hundred pounds a year. On the other hand, the elected Boards of Guardians were hard taskmasters, ever with an eye to saving ratepayers' money. Poor Law doctors found themselves saddled with gargantuan work loads. In 1836 Mr Wagstaffe of St Mary's, Lambeth, claimed in one year to have seen 6000 cases of illness, made 20,000 visits, and sent out 10,000 mixtures, 12,000 powders and 30,000 pills – and all on a salary of £105 a year [120]! Many received far less.

Another expedient increasingly common was to become a practitioner to the multitude of member-run friendly societies and benefit clubs that provided medical attention and medicines to working men, generally in return for contributions of a penny (1d.) a week. Once again, the assured income, if small, was an attractive prospect. But such a post generally meant a galling lack of autonomy. Above all, the friendly society doctor had to please his patients, otherwise a rival would appear at the end of the year, make a lower tender, and supplant him. When patients complained about their treatment, friendly society doctors were always liable to be hauled over the coals by the lay committee. Patient power and client control were, from the doctors' point of view, an unconscionable time a-dying [43].

Staking out a successful career thus involved a thorny path for the conscientious general practitioner in mid-Victorian England. He was a highly vulnerable individual in a competitive, buyers' market, in which it was not uncommon for doctors to undercut each other or to poach patients. Moreover, the medicine at his disposal was still little more effective than that possessed by his seventeenth-century counterparts: he would still be performing operations on the kitchen table or watching helplessly as babies died of summer diarrhoea, children succumbed to scarlet fever, and middle-aged patients to TB. Hence he had to work hard to keep the confidence of demanding and often disgruntled patients through being ever-ready to visit, generous with his time, and full of words of comfort: the classic bedside manner [117]. For an outsider, the prospects of rising up the profession to become a top consultant were negligible: such eminences still largely came from a self-selecting and -perpetuating elite.

In these circumstances it is hardly surprising that when in 1911 Lloyd George introduced his National Insurance scheme (whereby the state guaranteed medical treatment to contributing working men, through 'panel doctors' who would be paid an annual capita-tion fee by the state), the majority of practitioners joined the scheme, glad to have an assured income. The BMA huffed and puffed, fearing doctors would forfeit their independence, but a secure income counted for more. This situation was repeated after the Second World War with the setting up of the National Health Service. The BMA, the possibly unrepresentative mouthpiece of the GPs, was hostile: it feared that NHS doctors would be turned into state servants, reduced to the rank of post-office clerks. But that was not how it looked to many hard-up practitioners, plagued by prickly patients and the spectre of bad debts. For them the prospect of an annual fee per patient, paid by the state, seemed like a blessed release from insecurity. Many also had idealistic and political reasons for supporting the NHS. The vast majority of general practitioners had never had it so good as under the NHS [37; 124].

The nineteenth century thus produced a paradox. For the fortunes of rank-and-file practitioners remained precarious at pre-cisely the time when the state finally recognised the crucial importance to the nation's well-being of medicine and public health. Throughout Victoria's reign, a succession of scandals, revelations and reports uncovered appalling health risks, failures in the public provision of such elementary utilities as water and waste disposal, and mismanagement of medical services: many of these were the consequences of the staggering increase of slum housing, industrial pollution and occupational disease caused by a rocketing population and ultra-rapid industrialisation [137; 138]. The House of Commons Committees in 1807 and 1815 discovered barbarities in both public and private madhouses; the reports of the Poor Law Commissioners in the 1830s presented a welter of evidence proving that England's towns were death-traps for lack of adequate pure water, sanitation and sewage-disposal [15]. Factory inspectors' reports proved the workplace was a prime scene of disease, injury and accident. Successive visitations of cholera (the new plague) in 1831–2, 1848–9, 1854 and 1861, triggered urgent investigations of how filth, squalor and urban overcrowding combined to create perfect breeding-grounds for disease. Between them, Florence Nightingale and *The Times'* correspondent, William Russell, revealed grotesque hospital mismanagement in the Crimean War [120].

Awareness of terrible health hazards and medical shortcomings was nothing new. Back in the late-eighteenth century, the investigator and humanitarian John Howard had published two momentous works exposing the unhygienic conditions typical of hospitals and jails. Medical contemporaries of Howard, such as Lettsom, demonstrated how slums, overcrowding, urban filth and ignorance combined to create conditions ripe for lethal fever epidemics [11]. The point is that such revelations provoked almost no parliamentary response in the Georgian century. Following Howard, no Act of Parliament was passed instigating a general clean-up of prisons or inaugurating the removal of nuisances or slum clearance. In the nineteenth century, by contrast, airy new thoroughfares, like Charing Cross Road and Shaftesbury Avenue, would be bulldozed through the most pestiferous rookeries, courts and alleys. This is not to say that the Georgians were indifferent to welfare. Rather action was left to such local bodies as vestries and parishes and – an important new development – to semi-private, semi-public bodies of commissioners, who would undertake responsibility for street cleaning, refuse-disposal, lighting and so forth, in return for the power, secured by private Act of Parliament, to levy a rate. From the late-eighteenth century, such commissioners did good work in making most towns more habitable. They could not cope, however, with the sheer scale of the health risks of nineteenth-century conurbations.

For a variety of motives – necessity was one, the zeal of the utilitarian (Benthamite) and Evangelical lobbies another – the nineteenth-century state adopted a more interventionist role. The revelation of scandals generated public response, however delayed and deficient. Outcry over the evils of madhouses, for example, produced legislation in 1808 and 1845 setting up a nationwide system of public lunatic asylums, and Acts of 1828 and 1844 establishing the Lunacy Commissioners, a body whose job was to inspect madhouses and root out abuses [60]. Florence Nightingale's campaign led to a major reorganisation of military medical services and then of the nursing profession in general. The Board of Commissioners of the New Poor Law (1834), led by the indefatigable and dogmatic sanitarian, Edwin Chadwick, did much to alert the public to the unhealthiness of towns [37; 38]. Chadwick dedicated himself to a crusade against poverty; he believed much indigence was due to sickness, and maintained it was the state's duty to secure a healthier urban environment. The solution, in his view, lay in centralised powers to investigate the dangers caused by contaminated water, fetid cesspits, blocked drains, over-crowded churchyards and the like; and then to prosecute and legislate for improvements [34; 65; 139].

This is not the place to chronicle the growth of the public health services. But two trends should be mentioned. First, an infrastructure, however piecemeal, of medical and quasi-medical functionaries, and of public health institutions was being created from the 1830s, whose task was to safeguard the nation's welfare. Here the crucial development was the New Poor Law (1834). Not only did it make the workhouse the statutory mechanism for controlling England's growing army of paupers, but it set up alongside the workhouse the Poor Law infirmary. The diseases of the destitute, increasingly viewed as menacing the entire nation, were now too dangerous to be left to neighbourly self-help, private charity or *ad hoc* parish relief. Once established, Poor Law medical services expanded to meet the pressing needs their own existence had revealed and created. For example, fever and isolation hospitals were often added to workhouse wards, and non-paupers, suffering contagious diseases, were commonly removed to Poor Law infirmaries. In effect an NHS was being created for paupers a century before it was set up for the whole of society. Poor Law medicine, however, was characteristically cheeseparing, harsh and authoritarian, and was feared almost as much as the workhouse itself [1; 49].

Another crucial aspect of the creation of this public health infrastructure was the appointment of local Medical Officers of Health (MOsH), made possible by the Medical Act of 1848 and compulsory by an Act of 1872. Liverpool made the first appointment. John Simon (later Sir John) was appointed MOH for the City of London in 1848; other appointments followed [62; 82; 83]. A succession of Nuisance Removal Acts (1855, 1860, 1863) gave MOsH powers to regulate or eliminate such health threats as garbage tips, food adulteration, slaughterhouses, poisonous effluents and fumes. Once set up, their powers grew, both of investigation and prosecution. Georgian England had developed no equivalent of the 'medical police' bureaucracies common in Continental absolutist states. From the mid-nineteenth century, however, England at last had its 'medical policemen' [37; 112; 139].

Accompanying this permanent infrastructure went new public attitudes, above all the idea, fitfully but increasingly apparent, that the requirements of public health overrode sacred liberties of the person and of property. Reflecting on the cholera epidemic, *The Times* had pronounced in 1848 that it would rather take its chance with death than be bullied into health [31; 77; 88]. Such individualist, *laissez-faire* views gradually lost favour and were overtaken by events. In the 1840s, Parliament empowered the Board of Health through a series of statutes to act on such issues as polluted water supplies, contrary to the rights of the private water companies. That marked a major extension of central powers. In a similar way, legislation in 1853 eroded the liberty of the person and invaded the sanctuary of the family by making smallpox vaccination compulsory [62]. This was drastic action indeed, given that a sizeable minority of the population was, or was to become, violently opposed to vaccination, on grounds of science, religious faith and liberty. Slightly later, the Contagious Diseases Act (1867) continued the same trends. In an attempt to contain venereal disease in the British armed forces, Parliament empowered magistrates in stated garrison towns and ports to detain any woman suspected of being a prostitute; to subject her to medical examination; and, if found diseased, to force her to undergo compulsory medical treatment. This Act seemed to threaten individual liberty so dramatically, that it brought about an unlikely alliance of protests from old-style libertarians and new feminists [72].

By the time he came to write his eleventh annual report to the Privy Council in 1868, Sir John Simon could boast of the enlargement of the state's role:

It has interfered between parent and child, not only in imposing limitation on industrial uses of children, but also to the extent of requiring that children should not be left unvaccinated. It has interfered between employer and employed, to the extent of insisting, in the interests of the latter, that certain sanitary claims shall be fulfilled in all places of industrial occupation. It has interfered between vendor and purchaser; has put restrictions on the sale and purchase of poisons, has prohibited in certain cases certain commercial supplies of water, and has made it a public offence to sell adulterated food or drink or medicine, or to offer for sale any meat unfit for human food. Its care for the treatment of disease has not been unconditionally limited to treating at the public expense such sickness as may accompany destitution: it has provided that in any sort of epidemic emergency organized medical assistance, not peculiarly for paupers, may be required of local authorities; and in the same spirit it requires that vaccination at the public cost shall be given gratuitously to every claimant. [62]

From these public health developments it might seem that medicine was coming into its own, a knight in shining armour rescuing Britannia from the dragons of filth, cholera and other epidemics, environmental pollution, food adulteration and all the other health hazards produced by rampant population growth and unregulated market forces. At last the nation, it perhaps seemed, had recognised the true worth of the medical profession. Yet – and this is a second paradox – this is not what happened.

For the organised medical profession played a surprisingly ambivalent and often secondary role in the vast expansion of Victorian state health provision. Of course the work of hundreds of enlightened, humane practitioners throughout the nation in spotlighting the relations between squalor and disease and working for improvement cannot be gainsaid. In Manchester, for example,

James Kay-Shuttleworth proved an indefatigable activist, publishing in 1832 his classic *The Moral and Physical Condition of the Working Classes* [33; 90; 92]. Nevertheless, the Medical Colleges never gave a boost to the public health movement; similarly the pages of the *Lancet* echoed with the internal political squabbles of the profession rather than campaigning to improve the people's health. It is notable that neither of the two most vociferous and conspicuous champions of health, Edwin Chadwick and Florence Nightingale – both massively obstinate and immensely long-lived – was a doctor. That was, of course, true of Miss Nightingale by definition, because until the 1870s the medical profession's restrictive practices utterly debarred women from medicine. For his part, Chadwick was trained in the law, was a Prussian-style bureaucrat by temperament, and – perhaps more importantly – had done a stint as Jeremy Bentham's secretary [34; 65].

These two great public health champions were not only not doctors; they were, in many respects, positively anti-doctor. Chadwick in particular vilified the profession as supine and venal – a body (as they saw it) with such a vested interest in disease as to lack motivation for its eradication. For him the profession's primary involvement with clinical medicine, with treatment and cures, put the cart before the horse. Prevention was better than cure (not, thought Chadwick, that doctors were much good at curing, in any case!). But prevention could not be achieved so long as people were, perforce, living in a lethal environment [82; 83].

Chadwick, Nightingale and their supporters offered their own pet theories of health and disease. Chadwick liked to represent the medical profession as committed to the 'contagionist' hypothesis, that is the view that disease was spread through the transfer of disease 'seeds' by personal contact (a kind of precursor of Pasteur's germ theory). For Chadwick and like-minded sanitarians this was nonsense: for how was it that in epidemics, all people did not thereby 'catch' the disease? Instead Chadwick championed 'anti-contagionism' (as also did a fair percentage of doctors too), the view that sickness sprang from pestiferous 'miasmas', or contaminated atmospheres. Miasmas were bred and emitted by polluted water, sewage, animal ordure, industrial waste and the like: according to his pungent dictum, 'all smell is disease' [21; 88].

From this it followed that securing the public health hardly needed the mysterious art of the clinician. Rather, towns had to be cleaned up. For Chadwick and his supporters this meant the provision of two things: a plentiful pure-water supply, both for drinking and for flushing away waste, and a system of underground main drainage, to ensure that waste really was flushed out of towns, down to the sea or preferably to profit-making sewage farms, before it bred pestilence. So, public health hinged on engineering not medicine. In the mid-Victorian era, miracles of civil engineering set up the water and drainage system for London that is still essentially in place. Other cities followed suit. The death rate dropped. Although many individual doctors made distinguished contributions (for instance, John Snow's recognition that an outbreak of cholera in London's Soho stemmed from a poisoned pump), the professional bodies of the doctors remained bystanders. The relative indifference of the medical establishment to preventive, as distinct from curative, medicine, and to environmental and occupational medicine, is a legacy still with us today [112].

6
The role of medicine: what did it achieve?

In the last two chapters the rise of the medical profession has been traced from its comparatively unimportant status in Tudor and Stuart times. In the eighteenth century, it shared in the general expansion of a market economy. In the nineteenth century it achieved formal public blessing as a liberal profession and benefited from the state's growing involvement in public health with the progress of industrialization and urbanization.

But if medicine grew strong, did it actually promote health in others? After all, in *The Doctor's Dilemma* (1906), George Bernard Shaw could still present on the stage a bevy of top doctors shamelessly admitting to themselves (though not to their patients) that their medicine was bogus through and through. Lawrence Muggleton could opine in the seventeenth century: 'if there were never a doctor of physick in the world, people would live longer and live better in health'. Was such a view still tenable during the reign of Victoria [126]? And if so, how then do we explain its persistence?

The widest context against which to evaluate these questions is to ask whether medicine (of all sorts, from self-help to Harley Street, with public health thrown in as well) kept people alive. Did it have any significant effect upon the aggregate population? The death rate was strikingly high through most of the seventeenth century, peaking again in the 1720s and 30s, declining somewhat from the 1740s, rising again during the early nineteenth-century decades of rapid industrialisation. It began a slow but sustained decline from around 1830, and plummeted only in this century. Life expectancy, perhaps around 35 for males in the mid-seventeenth century, was around 40 by 1850 and had risen to 44 by 1890 [36; 141]. Today it is around 75.

The peaks and plateaux in the death rate were essentially due to mortality crises, caused by waves of epidemic disease, local or national, sporadic or sustained. Other major causes of death, like famine, important elsewhere in Europe, disappeared in England [2]. So the question is: when the death rate dipped, did medicine play a key role? Or, in more positive terms: did it play a part in the vast population rise gathering momentum from the 1740s and lasting throughout the period covered in this survey and beyond?

Today's leading historical demographers have convincingly argued that this sustained population growth stemmed not from a falling death-rate but primarily from a rising birth-rate. In its turn, the rising birth-rate is to be explained less by biological or medical factors than by social changes, above all, a trend towards earlier marriage amongst labouring people in an expansive economy typified by opportunity and insecurity [141].

Yet that still leaves the question of the possible role of medicine in bringing down mortality. There is scant evidence that medicine could do much throughout this entire period to counter the most lethal diseases. The plague was not conquered; it disappeared from Britain after 1666, but this had nothing to do with medicine, something to do with quarantine as imposed on a European scale [119], and perhaps most to do with the mysteries of epidemiology and the biohistory of rats and fleas. The same applies to cholera in the nineteenth century. It came; it conquered; it receded. Cleaner towns and water supplies had some impact, medicine none [31; 88]. Epidemics of typhus and dysentery caused mortality crises in the 1720s and 1730s: fevers seem to have proved less lethal in subsequent decades, possibly because immunity had been acquired or susceptibility reduced, but not because of any medical break-throughs in the strict sense. Not until the coming of the sulpha drugs in the 1930s and antibiotics like penicillin in the 1940s did medicine possess pharmaceutical means that would reliably save the lives of victims of infectious diseases [25]. In 1694 Queen Mary died of smallpox. As late as 1861, no less a personage than Prince Albert succumbed to typhoid.

Indeed, a distinguished medical professor, Thomas McKeown, has gone so far as to question 'the role of medicine' even in the very real and sustained fall in the death rate, a fall accelerating during Victoria's reign. Death claimed fewer victims, McKeown argues, not because medicine improved (hospitals, he suggests, 'positively did harm'), but mainly because of improved nutrition, made possible by rising standards of living which increased the nation's resistance. The environmental clean-up also played its part, McKeown believes [73].

The contrast McKeown draws between the roles of medicine and of engineering, nutrition and living standards is too extreme and artificial; and the current verdict upon hospitals is now more favourable; if they had really been 'gateways to death', it is hard to see why community and doctors alike continued to patronise them [140]. But, applied to the period from around 1650 to around 1850, McKeown's scepticism about medicine has some virtues. Medicine succeeded in making only marginal inroads into serious diseases. It scored one notable triumph. Between them, smallpox inoculation (introduced, be it remembered, by a lay woman) and vaccination (the work of Edward Jenner, a country doctor) diminished the terrors of a once-prevalent and commonly fatal disease, and so made some demographic contribution, not least because smallpox commonly left its survivors sterile. But what Razzell has called 'the conquest of smallpox' was matched by no equivalent conquest of any other major disease during the period covered by this book [104]. Medical science assuredly made its advances: Harvey discovered the circulation of the blood, William Hunter explained the lymphatic system, the workings of the nervous system were investigated, the physiology of respiration and digestion laid bare; but these advances in basic medical science could not quickly be translated into a therapeutic armoury, not least because the causes of disease and the nature of the body's morbid responses remained deeply obscure and fiercely contested. Advances in pathological anatomy, in cell science, basic physiology and organic chemistry, and the systematic observation of the sick *en masse* in hospitals did not bear significant fruit for saving lives till the last third of the nineteenth century and, above all, in the twentieth century. Modern surgery could not develop before the combination of anaesthetics and antiseptic (and later aseptic) conditions pioneered by Lister and others in the 1860s.

The fall in the death rate from the 1820s is hard to explain with confidence. It may have something to do with the life-cycle of infectious diseases, the immensely complicated interplay of humans, pathogens and environment. From about mid-century, however, better living standards and nutrition and improved sanitary conditions must take much credit [5; 7].

Does this mean that medicine was, and remained, Shaw's 'conspiracy', or at best a placebo offering psychological solace and hope (even if false hope) to those it could not grant cures? One should never, of course, despise the role of the doctor as drug, if that role is well acted. In a society in which, for complex reasons, the Christian clergy were ceasing to meet the personal needs of many – a society in which other comfort-giving professionals, such as social workers and psychiatric personnel, had not yet emerged – the trusted family doctor had much to contribute, through the confidences of the sick-bed, as friend, advisor and guide. Eighteenth- and nineteenth-century letters, diaries and fiction show that many practitioners were indeed admired and respected in such roles [91]. The family doctor frequently became a valued arbitrator and authority in domestic difficulties. Such authority might, of course, be double-edged. The doctor's say might convince a husband that it would be medically unwise for his wife to get pregnant again. On the other hand, as feminist scholars have rightly insisted, male-dominated medicine itself helped reinforce a vision of women as the weaker sex, incapable of responsibilities, exertion or even serious education, fit only for motherhood and domesticity. This belittling view blighted the lives of so many Victorian women [110].

But medicine was, in fact, far more than a placebo, or just a bedside manner. It could not vanquish the fatal diseases, but it could reduce pain, palliate discomfort, patch people up, and help them to cope with chronic disorders and disabilities – leg ulcers, abscesses, rheumatism, gout, dyspepsia and so forth. True, what the doctor ordered often differed little from what common sense dictated. The gout-ridden readily discovered for themselves that they hit the bottle at their peril. But the good clinician knew by training and experience how to manage such conditions as dropsy – severe and painful, though rarely immediately fatal – that might be completely beyond the know-how of the layman. Similarly, he was an invaluable surgeon who could set a fracture cleanly, or deliver a malpresented baby that had thwarted Nature and baffled the midwife's art.

This was the human face of medicine. But was medicine, as an organised profession, also more sinister? Radicals like Ivan Illich have argued that medicine today is indeed a conspiracy, in that it 'expropriates' health management from the people to the doctors, and 'medicalizes' life in the sense of asserting that many of the decisions respecting how we should run our affairs can be resolved only by medical experts [55]. Moreover, it is a 'con', because, so Illich contends, it creates more sickness than it cures.

Whatever the situation today, such an analysis hardly applies to early modern, or even to early industrial times. The medical profession had not then enveigled itself far into public life. It did not command a monopoly: it held few legal privileges: it was divided against itself. Unlike the other traditional professions – the law, the church and the army – it was barely an arm of state. Not least, lay medicine and client control of doctors remained widespread. Without the confident power of being able to conquer disease and tame death – a power that did not emerge till the present century – the doctor's place in society necessarily remained precarious.

Select bibliography

[1]   Abel-Smith, Brian (1964) *The Hospitals, 1800–1914* (London: Heinemann). A valuable survey, though concentrating mainly on administration and organisation.

[2]   Appleby, A. B. (1978) *Famine in Tudor and Stuart England* (Liverpool: Liverpool University Press). Convincingly shows that, in seventeenth-century England unlike much of the Continent, mortality crises were not a function of mass starvation.

[3]   Beier, L. M. (1987) *Sufferers and Healers: The Experience of Illness in Seventeenth-Century England* (London: Routledge & Kegan Paul). Examines health care from the viewpoint both of practitioners and patients.

[4]   Brewer, John and Porter, Roy (eds) (1992) *Consumption and the World of Goods* (London: Routledge). Essays examining the rise of commercial society since the eighteenth century.

[5]   Buer, M. C. (1926) *Health, Wealth, and Population in the Early Days of the Industrial Revolution* (London: G. Routledge & Sons). Despite its superseded demographic data, contains valuable discussion of eighteenth-century steps in the directions of public health and hygiene.

[6]   Burnby, J. G. L. (1983) *A Study of the English Apothecary from 1660 to 1760* (*Medical History*, Supplement 3). Presents abundant data to demonstrate that apothecaries existed in substantial numbers and shared advances in prosperity.

[7]   Burnett, J. (1966) *Plenty and Want: A Social History of Diet in England from 1815 to the Present Day* (London: Nelson). Highly readable survey of diet in context of changing standards of living, and its implications for health.

[8]   Bynum, W. F. (1980) 'Health, Disease and Medical Care', in G. S. Rousseau and R. Porter (eds), *The Ferment of Knowledge* (Cambridge: Cambridge University Press), 211–54. A lucid introduction to problems and the scholarly literature.

[9] Bynum, W. F. and Porter, Roy (eds) (1985) *William Hunter and the Eighteenth Century Medical World* (Cambridge: Cambridge University Press). Explorations of London medicine in the eighteenth century, including discussions of career structures, man-midwifery and medical education.

[10] Bynum, W. F. and Porter, Roy (eds) (1986) *Medical Fringe and Medical Orthodoxy 1750–1850* (London: Croom Helm). Analyses the changing relations between regular and irregular medicine in the context of medical professionalisation and the state.

[11] Bynum, W. F. and Porter, Roy (eds) (1991) *Living and Dying in London* (*Medical History*, Supplement 11, London: Wellcome Institute for the History of Medicine). Essays on mortality, morbidity and public health.

[12] Bynum, W. F. and Porter, Roy (eds) (1993) *The Routledge Companion Encyclopaedia of the History of Medicine* (London: Routledge). The most comprehensive introduction to the history of medicine.

[13] Cameron, H. C. (1954) *Mr Guy's Hospital, 1726–1948* (London, New York and Toronto: Longmans Green). Brings out the importance of personal philanthropy in the development of the English hospital system.

[14] Cartwright, F. F. (1977) *A Social History of Medicine* (London: Longman). Though highly compressed and selective, this represents the best attempt yet to place medical transformations in their social context.

[15] [Chadwick, Edwin] (1974) *The Poor Law Report of 1834*, S. G. and O. A. Checkland (eds) (Harmondsworth: Penguin). The most influential official publication for changing attitudes to public health published in the nineteenth century, reprinted with a useful introduction.

[16] Chapman, Stanley (1973) *Jesse Boot of Boots the Chemists* (London: Hodder & Stoughton). Demonstrates how Boots the Chemists had its origins in the Victorian medical fringe.

[17] Clark, Sir George (1964, 1966, 1972) *A History of the Royal College of Physicians of London*, 3 vols (Oxford: Clarendon Press). The standard official history of the College, packed with facts, rather bland in tone.

[18] Clark-Kennedy, Archibald E. (1979) *London Pride: The Story of a Voluntary Hospital* (London: Hutchinson Benham). A well-researched account of the London, one of the new voluntary hospitals of the Georgian age.

[19] Clarkson, Leslie (1975) *Death, Disease and Famine in Pre-Industrial England* (Dublin: Gill and Macmillan). Illuminating analysis of the interplay between social and biological forces in the patterns of

morbidity and mortality, valuable for making sense of more strictly demographic sources, such as [141].

[20] Cook, Harold J. (1986) *The Decline of the Old Medical Regime in Stuart London* (Ithaca: Cornell University Press). Examines the politics of London medicine in the seventeenth century, especially the declining fortunes of the College of Physicians. Good counterbalance to Webster [133].

[21] Cooter, R. (1982) 'Anticontagionism and History's Medical Record', in P. Wright and A. Treacher (eds), *The Problem of Medical Knowledge* (Edinburgh: Edinburgh University Press), pp. 87–108. Illuminating exploration of the intertwining of theories of disease with social, moral and political attitudes.

[22] Cope, Sir Zachary (1966) 'The Private Medical Schools of London 1874–1914', in Poynter, F. N. L. (ed.), *The Evolution of Medical Education in Britain* (London: Pitman), pp. 89–109. Shows the important role played by private institutions in the rise of English medical education.

[23] Cope, Sir Vincent Zachary (1959) *The History of the Royal College of Surgeons of England* (London: Anthony Blond). Useful, but 'official' in its outlook. The College is due for fresh historical interpretation.

[24] Copeman, W. S. C. (1967) *The Worshipful Society of Apothecaries of London. A History 1617–1967* (Oxford: Pergamon Press). Correctly emphasises the role of the Society as a trade guild.

[25] Creighton, Charles (1965) *A History of Epidemics in Britain*, 2 vols (Cambridge: Cambridge University Press, 1st edn, 1891–4). A massive compilation, unreliable in individual detail, but still of great value for its abundance of evidence.

[26] Cunningham, Andrew, and French, Roger (eds) (1990) *The Medical Enlightenment of the Eighteenth Century* (Cambridge: Cambridge University Press). A valuable collection of scholarly essays on eighteenth-century medicine.

[27] Curtin, Philip D. (1989) *Death by Migration: Europe's Encounter with the Tropical World in the Nineteenth Century* (Cambridge and New York: Cambridge University Press). A well researched investigation of attempts to fight tropical diseases within the British Empire.

[28] Dainton, Courtney (1961) *The Story of England's Hospitals* (London: Museum Press). In the absence of full scholarly survey of the rise of hospitals, this rather slight work still has some value.

[29] Digby, Anne (1985) *Madness, Morality and Medicine. A Study of the York Retreat, 1796–1914* (Cambridge: Cambridge University Press). Fully-researched and penetrating analysis of the workings of England's leading private lunatic asylum, especially welcome for its emphasis upon patients.

[30]   Donnison, Jean (1977) *Midwives and Medical Men: A History of Interprofessional Rivalries and Women's Rights* (London: Heinemann Educational). A powerfully written account of how men came to replace women from the late seventeenth century onwards as the providers of obstetrical services.

[31]   Durey, M. (1979) *The Return of the Plague: British Society and the Cholera 1831–2* (Dublin: Gill and Macmillan). Admirable analysis of social, moral and political responses to cholera.

[32]   Ehrenreich, Barbara and English, Deirdre (1974) *Complaints and Disorders: The Sexual Politics of Sickness* (New York: Old Westbury). A spirited statement of the feminist case that medicine has contributed to the social control of women.

[33]   Eyler, J. M. (1979) *Victorian Social Medicine. The Ideas and Methods of William Farr* (Baltimore: Johns Hopkins University Press). An intelligent and sympathetic intellectual biography of the leading medical statistician of Victorian England, showing how data helped awaken the public conscience.

[34]   Finer, S. E. (1952) *Life and Times of Edwin Chadwick* (London: Methuen). Superb biography of the foremost public health campaigner, with an intelligent assessment of the importance of Chadwick's utilitarian background.

[35]   Fissell, Mary E. (1991) *Patients, Power and the Poor in Eighteenth-Century Bristol* (Cambridge: Cambridge University Press). A well-researched regional study of the interlocking of poverty, the Poor Law and medical services, especially illuminating on the role of hospitals.

[36]   Flinn, Michael W. (1981) *The European Demographic System 1500–1820* (Brighton, Sussex: Harvester Press). Powerful overview of how Europe as a whole broke out of the biological '*ancien régime*'. Good on the comparative dimension.

[37]   Fraser, D. (1973) *The Evolution of the British Welfare State. A History of Social Policy since the Industrial Revolution* (London: Macmillan). A well-digested and balanced survey of the growing role of the state in providing public health and welfare. Sensitive to questions of interpretation.

[38]   Frazer, W. M. (1950) *A History of English Public Health, 1833–1939* (London: Baillière). A solid, factual account.

[39]   French, Roger and Wear, Andrew (eds) (1989) *The Medical Revolution of the Seventeenth Century* (Cambridge and New York: Cambridge University Press). New research findings, emphasizing continuity as well as change.

[40]   French, Roger and Wear, Andrew (eds) (1991) *British Medicine in an Age Of Reform* (London: Routledge). A collection of essays focusing on the first half of the nineteenth century, and under-

lining the links between medicine and the broader scientific movement.

[41]   Gittings, Clare (1984) *Death, Burial and the Individual in Early
Modern England* (London: Croom Helm). Provides insights into
attitudes towards death, which the author treats as an increasingly
'individual' experience.

[42]   Granshaw, Lindsay and Porter, Roy (eds) (1989) *The Hospital in
History* (London: Routledge; paperback edition, 1990). A collection
of essays which show how the hospital developed an increasing
medical profile and function.

[43]   Green, David G. (1985) *Working Class Patients and the Medical
Establishment. Self-Help in Britain from the Mid-nineteenth Century to
1948* (London: Gower/Maurice Temple Smith). A sympathetic
exploration of the health care provisions offered by friendly societies.

[44]   Hamilton, B. (1951) 'The Medical Professions in the Eighteenth
Century', *Economic History Review*, 2nd series, iv, 141–69. Though
dated, still a valuable account of the structuring of the medical
professions. To be used together with the work of Lane, Loudon
and Waddington.

[45]   Hamilton, D. (1981) *The Healers: A History of Medicine in Scotland*
(Edinburgh: Canongate). Brings out the special contribution of the
Scots to British medicine, in particular the scientific education
provided from early times by Edinburgh and then Glasgow universities.

[46]   Helman, Cecil (1984) *Culture, Health and Illness* (Bristol: John
Wright). Stimulating exploration of the meanings of health and
disease, and the symbolic significance of therapies, from the viewpoint of the sick person and the community.

[47]   Hembry, Phyllis (1990) *The English Spa 1560–1815: A Social
History* (London: Althone Press). Particularly underlines the
double role of the spa as medical centre and leisure resort.

[48]   Hobhouse, Edmund (1934) *The Diary of a West Country Physician,
AD 1684–1726* (London: Simpkin Marshall). Reveals the medical
practice of Claver Morris, a practitioner from Wells.

[49]   Hodgkinson, Ruth G. (1967) *The Origins of the National Health
Service: The Medical Services of the New Poor Law, 1834–1871*
(London: Wellcome Historical Medical Library, London). Very
fully documented account of the rise of the Poor Law medical
service, following the New Poor Law of 1834.

[50]   Holloway, S. W. F. (1964) 'Medical Education in England, 1833–
1858: A Sociological Analysis', *History*, xlix, 299–324. Demonstrates that debates over the quality of medical education reflected
deep divisions within the medical profession about its own structure.

[51] Holloway, S. W. F. (1966) 'The Apothecaries' Act of 1815: A Reinterpretation', 2 parts, *Medical History*, x, 107–29; and x, 221–36. A major revisionist discussion, arguing that the apothecaries probably lost more than they gained by the Act of 1815, and thus showing the strength of the old hierarchy.

[52] Holloway, S. W. F. (1991) *Royal Pharmaceutical Society of Great Britain 1841–1991* (London: The Pharmaceutical Press). Much wider than the title suggests: now the best general survey of the history of British pharmacy.

[53] Houlbrooke, Ralph (ed.) (1989) *Death, Ritual and Bereavement* (London: Routledge). A collection of essays placing death in its medical, religious, cultural and social settings.

[54] Hultin, N. C. (1975) 'Medicine and Magic in the Eighteenth Century: the Diaries of James Woodforde', *Journal of the History of Medicine and Allied Sciences*, xxx, 349–66. Fascinating account of the 'magical' remedies used by the mid-eighteenth century parson.

[55] Illich, I. (1978) *The Limits of Medicine* (Harmondsworth: Penguin Books). Primarily a polemic, though with a historical dimension, denouncing the alleged rise of modern medical dependency, and the medical profession's part in fostering that dependence.

[56] Inglis, Brian (1964) *Fringe Medicine* (London: Faber & Faber). An enterprising attempt to trace the roots of the modern medical fringe. Use in connection with [10].

[57] Jewson, N. (1974) 'Medical Knowledge and the Patronage System in Eighteenth Century England', *Sociology*, xii, 369–85. Argues rather schematically that traditional medicine, both as social practice and as scientific theory, depended heavily upon the influence wielded by aristocratic patients.

[58] Jewson N. (1976) 'The Disappearance of the Sick Man from Medical Cosmology, 1770–1870', *Sociology*, x, 225–44. A subtle analysis of the changes made by the rise of physical diagnosis and the development of scientific medicine.

[59] Johnson, T. J. (1972) *Professions and Power* (London and Basingstoke: Macmillan). Argues against the 'altruistic' view of professions, seeing them as dedicated to gaining quasi-monopolistic powers for their members.

[60] Jones, Kathleen (1972) *A History of the Mental Health Services* (London and Boston: Routledge & Kegan Paul). Important if rather idealistic account of the state's growing involvement with mental health.

[61] Keevil, J. J. (1957–63) *Medicine and the Navy 1200–1900* (vol. 1, 1200–1649, vol. 2, 1649–1714) (Edinburgh and London: Livingstone). A massive and well-documented history. See also [67].

[62] Lambert, R. (1963) *Sir John Simon 1816–1904 and English Social*

Administration (London: MacGibbon and Kee). The authoritative biography of the most important medical officer of the state in the nineteenth century.

[63] Lane, Joan (1984) 'The Medical Practitioners of Provincial England in 1783', *Medical History*, xxviii, 353–71. Important analysis of the structure of provincial practice in the late eighteenth century.

[64] Lewis, J. S. (1986) *In the Family Way: Childbearing in the British Aristocracy 1760–1860* (New Brunswick, N.J.: Rutgers University Press). The best account of changing birthing practices, emphasizing the new fashion for the use of the man-midwife.

[65] Lewis, R. A. (1952) *Edwin Chadwick and the Public Health Movement 1832–1854* (London: Longmans Green). Relates Chadwick's life to the growing public concern about health matters.

[66] Llewellyn, Nigel (1991) *The Art of Death* (London: Reaktion Books). A well-illustrated survey of the culture of dying in early modern England.

[67] Lloyd, C. and Coulter, J. S. L. (1961–3) *Medicine and the Navy 1200–1900* (vol. 3, 1714–1815, vol. 4, 1815–1900) (Edinburgh and London: Livingstone). A massive and standard history. See also [61].

[68] Loudon, Irvine S. (1981) 'The Origins and Growth of the Dispensary Movement in England', *Bulletin of the History of Medicine*, iv, 322–42. Examines the dispensary movement as one of the roots of public health concern.

[69] Loudon, Irvine S. (1987) *Medical Care and the General Practitioner, 1750–1850* (Oxford: Oxford University Press). A fundamentally important account of the emergence of the family doctor.

[70] McClure, Ruth (1981) *Coram's Children* (New Haven, Connecticut, and London: Yale University Press). A well-researched account of London's main orphanage, arguing that it was efficiently and humanely managed.

[71] McGrew, Roderick E. (1985) *Encyclopedia of Medical History* (London: Macmillan). A reliable reference work on the history of medical theory and practice, paying special attention to diseases.

[72] McHugh, Paul (1980) *Prostitution and Victorian Social Reform* (London: Croom Helm). A fine study of the Contagious Diseases Act.

[73] McKeown, Thomas (1976) *The Modern Rise of Population* (London: Edward Arnold). McKeown casts doubt on the idea that medical progress produced diminished mortality. Nutrition and (to a lesser degree) environmental factors instead are stressed.

[74] McLaren, A. (1984) *Reproductive Rituals* (New York: Methuen). A pioneering survey of popular attitudes and practices regarding pregnancy, reproduction and infanticide.

[75] Matthew, Leslie G. (1962) *History of Pharmacy in Britain* (Edinburgh and London: Livingstone). Useful narrative account.

[76] Miller, G. (1957) *The Adoption of Inoculation for Smallpox in England and France* (London: Oxford University Press). Shows the importance of social and political factors in the speedier adoption of inoculation in Britain.

[77] Morris, R. J. (1976) *Cholera, 1832* (London: Croom Helm). Particularly interesting on the relative impact – both physical and mental – of cholera on different classes of society.

[78] Moscucci, Ornella (1990) *The Science of Woman: Gynaecology and Gender in England, 1800–1929* (Cambridge: Cambridge University Press). An important investigation of the treatment of women within nineteenth-century medicine.

[79] Mullett, Charles (1946) 'Public Baths and Health in England, 16th–18th century', *Bulletin of the History of Medicine*, Supplement No. 5 (Baltimore). By showing the traditional importance of public baths, Mullett undermines the popular notion that cleanliness was a nineteenth-century invention.

[80] Nagy, Doreen Evenden (1988) *Popular Medicine in Seventeenth-Century England* (Ohio: Bowling Green State University Popular Press). A sensible survey of traditional healing practices.

[81] Newman, Charles (1957) *The Evolution of Medical Education in the 19th Century* (London: Oxford University Press). The standard account of the emergence of the modern teaching hospital.

[82] Newham, George (1932) *The Rise of Preventive Medicine* (Oxford: Oxford University Press). Surveys the concept of prevention from Antiquity onwards.

[83] Newsholme, Sir Arthur (1927) *Evolution of Preventive Medicine* (Baltimore: Williams & Wilkins). Though dated, contains an important insider's account of the role increasingly played by the state in public health.

[84] Nutton, Vivian and Porter, Roy (eds) (1993) *History of Medical Education in Britain* (Amsterdam: Rodopi). The most up-to-date account of the training of doctors.

[85] Owen, David (1965) *English Philanthropy 1660–1940* (Cambridge, Massachusetts: Belknap Press). Demonstrates the importance of charity and humanitarianism in the growth of medical facilities in England.

[86] Oxley, G. W. (1974) *Poor Relief in England and Wales 1601–1834* (Newton Abbot: David and Charles). A clear, brief guide to the workings of the Old Poor Law.

[87] Parry-Jones, William (1972) *The Trade in Lunacy. A Study of Private Madhouses in England in the Eighteenth and Nineteenth Centuries* (London: Routledge & Kegan Paul). Shows, through a wealth of

detail, the importance of private provision in the emergence of care for the mentally ill.

[88]   Pelling, M. (1978) *Cholera, Fever and English Medicine 1825–1865* (Oxford: Oxford University Press). Particularly strong on the alternative medical theories for understanding and combating cholera.

[89]   Peterson, M. J. (1978) *The Medical Profession in Mid-Victorian London* (Berkeley: University of California Press). The best account of the emergence of the modern British medical profession, stressing the importance of specialisation, the teaching hospitals and the rise of Harley Street in the early Victorian age.

[90]   Pickstone, John V. (1985) *Medicine and Industrial Society. A History of Hospital Development in Manchester and its Region 1752–1946* (Manchester: Manchester University Press). An insightful account of the part played by voluntary and municipal hospitals in the life of new industrial communities.

[91]   Porter, Dorothy and Porter, Roy (1989) *Patient's Progress: Doctors and Doctoring in Eighteenth-Century England* (Cambridge: Polity Press). Examines the interplay of patients and doctors.

[92]   Porter, Dorothy and Porter, Roy (eds) (1993) *Doctors, Politics and Society* (Amsterdam: Rodopi). A series of essays investigating the interface between doctors, parliament and the state.

[93]   Porter, Roy (ed.) (1985) *Patients and Practitioners. Lay Perceptions of Medicine in Pre-Industrial Society* (Cambridge: Cambridge University Press). Essays examining how sick people coped with disease – and with their doctors.

[94]   Porter, Roy (1985) 'The Patient's View: Doing Medical History from Below', *Theory and Society*, xiv, 175–98. States the priorities of a patient-centred social history of medicine.

[95]   Porter, Roy (1987) *Mind Forg'd Manacles: Madness and Psychiatry in England from Restoration to Regency* (London: Athlone Press; paperback edition, Penguin, 1990). A study of the treatment of the insane in eighteenth-century England.

[96]   Porter, Roy and Porter, Dorothy (1988) *In Sickness and in Health: The British Experience 1650–1850* (London: Fourth Estate). Examines the 'sickness culture' of eighteenth-century England, emphasizing the active role of the laity in managing their own health.

[97]   Porter, Roy (1989) *Health for Sale: Quackery in England 1650–1850* (Manchester: Manchester University Press). A study of fringe medicine that stresses its parallels with regular medicine and its integration into a commercial economy.

[98]   Porter, Roy (1991) *Doctor of Society: Thomas Beddoes and the Sick Trade in Late Enlightenment England* (London: Routledge). The life

of a physician who was both a political radical and a violent critic of his own profession.

[99] Porter, Roy (ed.) (1992) *The Popularization of Medicine, 1650–1850* (London: Routledge). A collection of essays about the role of literacy and popular books in spreading medical knowledge.

[100] Pound, Reginald (1967) *Harley Street* (London: Michael Joseph). Anecdotal but informative.

[101] Poynter, F. N. L. (ed.) (1966) *The Evolution of Medical Education in Britain* (London: Pitman). Essays looking at the variety of forms of medical education, including apprenticeship.

[102] Poynter, F. N. L. (ed.) (1964) *The Evolution of Hospitals in Britain* (London: Pitman). Essays examining the diverse forms of hospital provision in England, both public and private, general and specialised.

[103] Ramsey, Matthew (1988) *Professional and Popular Medicine in France, 1770–1830* (New York: Cambridge University Press). An excellent survey of the relations in France between medicine and the state.

[104] Razzell, Peter (1975) *The Conquest of Smallpox* (Firle, Sussex: Caliban Press). Argues that the work of Jenner has been misinterpreted and overrated, and shows that inoculation was relatively safe and an important life-saver.

[105] Richardson, Ruth (1987) *Death, Dissection and the Destitute: A Political History of the Human Corpse* (London: Routledge & Kegan Paul). A moving study of popular resistance to medical dissection in the era of Burke and Hare.

[106] Riley, James C. (1986) *The Eighteenth-Century Campaign to Avoid Disease* (London: Macmillan). Important new study of early preventive medicine.

[107] Riley, James C. (1989) *Sickness, Recovery and Death: A History and Forecast of Ill Health* (Iowa City: University of Iowa Press; London: Macmillan; Houndmills, Basingstoke, Hampshire: Macmillan). Riley argues that growing life expectations have entailed the rise of new sicknesses.

[108] Risse, Guenter (1986) *Hospital Life in Enlightenment Scotland: Care and Teaching at the Royal Infirmary of Edinburgh* (Cambridge: Cambridge University Press). Our fullest study of an eighteenth-century hospital, with copious detail on both the patients and their conditions.

[109] Roberts, David (1960) *Victorian Origins of the British Welfare State* (New Haven: Yale University Press). Broad and sympathetic account of state intervention in the Victorian age.

[110] Roberts, R. (ed.) (1981) *Women, Health and Reproduction* (London: Routledge & Kegan Paul). Essays mainly from a feminist point of

view, showing that the rise of modern, male-dominated medicine is
a mixed blessing for women.

[111] Roberts, R. S. (1962, 1964) 'The Personnel and Practice of
Medicine in Tudor and Stuart England', *Medical History*, vi, 363–
82; vii, 217–34. A pioneering survey. Use with [132].

[112] Rosen, George (1958) *A History of Public Health* (New York: MD
Publications). The major survey of the history of public health on
an international plane.

[113] Rosner, Lisa (1990) *Medical Education in the Age of Improvement:
Edinburgh Students and Apprentices 1760–1826* (Edinburgh: Edinburgh University Press). A well-researched account of the development of medical education in Edinburgh.

[114] Russell, Andrew W. (ed.) (1981) *The Town and State Physician in
Europe from the Middle Ages to the Enlightenment* (Wolfenbüttel:
Herzog August Bibliothek). Essays examining the civic roots of the
public health movement in many European countries.

[115] Schupbach, William (1985) 'Sequah: An English "American Med-
icine-Man" in 1890', *Medical History*, xxix, 272–317. Vivid account
of a late nineteenth-century quack.

[116] Shorter, Edward (1982) *A History of Women's Bodies* (London:
Allen Lane). A controversial history which seeks to establish the
benefits which modern medicine has brought to women, in particular through reducing childbirth mortality.

[117] Shorter, Edward (1986) *Bedside Manners* (Harmondsworth: Allen
Lane). A brisk history, covering America, Britain and Europe, of
the changing status of the general practitioner.

[118] Slack, Paul (1980) 'Books of Orders: The Making of English Social
Policy, 1577–1631', *Transactions of the Royal Historical Society*, 5th
Series, xxx, 1–22. Examines provision for health as part of a
broader emergence of social policy.

[119] Slack, Paul (1985) *The Impact of Plague in Tudor and Stuart England*
(London: Routledge & Kegan Paul). A major account of responses,
political, social, medical and religious, to the great scourge of the
sixteenth and seventeenth centuries. Argues that more effective
measures emerged slowly in Britain.

[120] Smith, F. B. (1979) *The People's Health 1830–1910* (London:
Croom Helm). Statistically-rich investigations of the state of the
nation's health in the nineteenth century; short on interpretation.

[121] Sprigge, S. Squire (1899) *The Life and Times of Thomas Wakley,
Founder and First Editor of the 'Lancet', Member of Parliament for
Finsbury and Coroner for West Middlesex* (London: Longmans,
Green and Co.). The best biography of one of the key medical
campaigners and reformers of the nineteenth century.

[122] Starr. P. (1982) *The Social Transformation of American Medicine*

(New York: Basic Books). A sociologically-oriented interpretation of the changing place of doctors in American society.

[123] Suzuki, Akihito (1991, 1992) 'Lunacy in Seventeenth- and Eighteenth-Century England: Analysis of Quarter Sessions Records', *History of Psychiatry*, ii, 437–56; iii, 29–44. This article demonstrates that, before 1750, most English lunatics were treated at home or by the parish.

[124] Thane, P. (1982) *The Foundations of the Welfare State* (London: Longman). Clear and balanced account.

[125] Thomas, E. G. (1980) 'The Old Poor Law and Medicine', *Medical History*, xxiv, 1–19. Shows that the Old Poor Law was quite generous in its medical provisions.

[126] Thomas, Keith (1971) *Religion and the Decline of Magic. Studies in Popular Beliefs in Sixteenth- and Seventeenth-Century England* (London: Weidenfeld and Nicolson). Contains a wealth of material on popular medicine and its connections to magic and witchcraft.

[127] Turner, E. S. (1958) *Call the Doctor: A Social History of Medical Men* (London: Michael Joseph). A lively, entertaining narrative.

[128] Versluysen, Margaret Connor (1981) 'Midwives, Medical Men and "Poor Women Labouring of Child"; Lying-in Hospitals in Eighteenth Century London', in H. Roberts (ed.), *Women, Health and Reproduction* (London: Routledge & Kegan Paul), 18–49. Important interpretation of the effects for women of the emergence of maternity hospitals in the eighteenth century.

[129] Waddington, Ivan (1973) 'The Struggle to Reform the Royal College of Physicians, 1767–1771: A Sociological Analysis', *Medical History*, xvi, 107–26. Demonstrates the entrenchment of the old medical hierarchy.

[130] Waddington, Ivan (1984) *The Medical Profession in the Industrial Revolution* (Dublin: Gill and Macmillan). A mature and well-organised sociological account of the 'modernization' of the medical profession, discounting any simple theory of 'progress'.

[131] Wear, Andrew (ed.) (1992) *Medicine in Society: Historical Essays* (Cambridge/New York: Cambridge University Press). The best broad survey of the social dimension of medical developments.

[132] Webster, Charles (ed.) (1979) *Health, Medicine and Mortality in the Sixteenth Century* (Cambridge: Cambridge University Press). Essays full of informative research relating to the early modern medical profession.

[133] Webster, Charles (1975) *The Great Instauration. Science, Medicine and Reform, 1626–1660* (London: Duckworth). The best account of attempts (mainly 'Puritan') to reform medicine in the seventeenth century, showing how the Restoration of 1660 led to their failure.

[134] Weindling, Paul (ed.) (1985) *The Social History of Occupational*

Health (London: Croom Helm). A major account of job-related disease and the rise of occupational medicine.

[135] Williams, G. (1981) *The Age of Miracles. Medicine and Surgery in the Nineteenth Century* (London: Constable). A popular history of nineteenth-century medicine.
[136] Williams, G. (1975) *The Age of Agony: The Art of Healing c.1700–1800* (London: Constable). A popular account of eighteenth-century medicine.
[137] Wohl, Anthony S. (1977) *The Eternal Slum. Housing and Social Policy in Victorian London* (London: Edward Arnold). Shows how revelations of unhealthy living conditions led to urban reform.
[138] Wohl, Anthony S. (1983) *Endangered Lives. Public Health in Victorian Britain* (London: Dent). A fine analysis of the part played by medical men in the generation of public health agitation.
[139] Woods, Robert and Woodward, John (1984) *Urban Disease and Mortality in Nineteenth Century England* (London: Batsford). Valuable essays integrating urban history, historical demography and medical history.
[140] Woodward, John (1974) *To Do the Sick No Harm. A Study of the British Voluntary Hospital System to 1875* (London and Boston: Routledge & Kegan Paul). A valuable history of the voluntary hospital movement.
[141] Wrigley, E. A. and Schofield, R. S. (1981) *The Population History of England, 1541–1871. A Reconstruction* (London: Edward Arnold). The authoritative source for English demographic history, though it has relatively little to say on the medical dimensions of morbidity and mortality.

The recently published work by Anne Digby, *Making a Medical Living: Doctors and Patients in the English Market for Medicine, 1720–1911* (Cambridge: Cambridge University Press, 1994), is the first detailed exploration of the economics of medical practice in England in this period. It tends to confirm Loudon's view that the eighteenth century was a golden age for the practitioner, whereas the nineteenth century brought periods when doctors flooded the market and so enjoyed reduced economic prospects.

Index

anaesthetics 61
antiseptics 61
apothecaries 12, 28
Apothecaries, Society of 12, 49
  Apothecaries Act (1815) 46
Arnold, Thomas 39
asylums 31, 38–40

Bacon, Francis 6
Baillie, Matthew 35, 36
Barber Surgeons Company 12
Baxter, Richard 18, 22
Bentham, Jeremy and Benthamites
  54
Board of Health 55
Boot, Jesse 43
British Medical Association 49, 52

Chadwick, Edwin 54, 57–8
cholera 55, 60
Contagious Diseases Act (1867)
  55

Darwin, Erasmus 36
death, 21; death rate 59–62
Dell, William 5
Dimsdale, Thomas 37
dispensaries 32
drugs 7–8

empirics 13, 14
epidemics 20, 32, 60

Fothergill, John 28

Galen 5, 7
Garth, Samuel 36
General Medical Council 49
general practitioners 29, 50–2, 62
Greatrakes, Valentine 14–15

Harvey, William 27
Heberden, William 35
herbalism 42
hospitals 15–16, 30–3, 61
  maternity 31–2
Howard, John 53
humours 19
Hunter, William 28, 35, 36, 38, 61

incomes 36
inoculation 37
insanity 15

James, Robert, and his Fever
  Powders 43
Jenner, Edward 61
Johnson, Samuel 24, 43
Josselin, Ralph 13, 22

Kay-Shuttleworth, Sir James 56

Lancet 45
Lettsom, J. C. 28, 35, 36
lunatic asylums 31, 38–40

magic 21
Mead, Richard 35, 36
Medical education; Oxford and
    Cambridge, 6, 29; in hospitals,
    34; private anatomy schools, 42;
    at new universities 50
medical insurance 34
'medical model' 19
Medical Officers of Health 55
'medicalisation' 44
miasmas 20, 57
midwifery 30, 32, 40
Montagu, Elizabeth 25
Montagu, Lady Mary Wortley 37
mortality crises 60

mountebanks 14
Muggleton, Lodowick 5

National Health Service 6, 35
National Insurance scheme (1911)
    52
naval medicine 29
New Poor Law (1834) 54
Nightingale, Florence 53, 57
Norwich, medicine in 12, 13

obstetricians 30, 37, 40
orphanages 32

Paracelsus 5, 7, 8
Pepys, Samuel 7, 8, 18, 22, 23
Percival, Dr Thomas 25
physic 11
plague 6, 9, 22
Poor Law medicine 16, 37
population levels 59
Pringle, John 37
public health 52, 54

quacks 14, 25, 40–1

religion and medicine 21–2

Royal College of Physicians 5, 12, 27,
    49
Royal Humane Society 35
Royal Society of London 27

sanitary reform 53, 57–8
self-medication 23
'Sequah' (quack doctor) 41
Shaw, George Bernard 25, 59, 62
Simon, Sir John 55, 56
Sloane, Sir Hans 35
Smollett, Tobias 36
Solomon, Samuel 41
surgeons 11
Surgeons' Company 28
    Surgeons' College 47
surgery 8, 28, 61
Sydenham, Thomas 27

therapeutics 7, 40, 42, 62
typhus 7

Wakley, Thomas 45
Ward, Joshua 41, 43
Wentworth, Thomas 9
Willis, Revd Dr Francis 39
witchcraft 21

New Studies in Economic and Social History

Titles in the series available from Cambridge University Press:

1. M. Anderson
    Approaches to the history of the Western family, 1500–1914

2. W. Macpherson
    The economic development of Japan, 1868–1941

3. R. Porter
    Disease, medicine, and society in England: second edition

4. B.W.E. Alford
    British economic performance since 1945

5. A. Crowther
    Social policy in Britain, 1914–1939

6. E. Roberts
    Women's work 1840–1940

7. C. O'Grada
    The great Irish famine

8. R. Rodger
    Housing in urban Britain 1780–1914

9. P. Slack
    The English Poor Law 1531–1782

10. J.L. Anderson
    Explaining long-term economic change

11. D. Baines
    Emigration from Europe 1815–1930

12. M. Collins
    Banks and industrial finance 1800–1939

13. A. Dyer
    Decline and growth in English towns 1400–1640

14. R.B. Outhwaite
    Dearth, public policy and social disturbance in England, 1550–1800

15. M. Sanderson
    Education, economic change and society in England

16. R.D. Anderson
    Universities and elites in Britain since 1800

17. C. Heywood
    The development of the French economy, 1700–1914

18. R.A. Houston
    The population history of Britain and Ireland 1500–1750

19. A.J. Reid
    Social classes and social relations in Britain 1850–1914

20. R. Woods
    The population of Britain in the nineteenth century

21. T.C. Barker
    The rise of road transport, 1700–1990

22. J. Harrison
    The Spanish economy

23. C. Schmitz
    The growth of big business in the United States and Western Europe, 1850–1939

24. R.A. Church
    The rise and decline of the British motor industry

25. P. Horn
    Children's work and welfare, 1780–1880

26. R. Perren
    Agriculture in depression, 1870–1940

27. R.J. Overy
    The Nazi economic recovery 1932–1938: second edition

Previously published as

Studies in Economic History

Titles in the series available from the Macmillan Press Limited

1. B.W.E. Alford
   Depression and recovery? British economic growth, 1918–1939

2. M. Anderson
   Population change in north-western Europe, 1750–1850

3. S.D. Chapman
   The cotton industry in the industrial revolution: second edition

4. N. Charlesworth
   British rule and the Indian economy, 1800–1914

5. L.A. Clarkson
   Proto-industrialisation: the first phase of industrialisation

6. D.C. Coleman
   Industry in Tudor and Stuart England

7. I.M. Drummond
   The gold standard and the international monetary system, 1900–1939

8. M.E. Falkus
   The industrialisation of Russia, 1700–1914

9. J.R. Harris
   The British iron industry, 1700–1850

10. J. Hatcher
    Plague, population and the English economy, 1348–1530

11. J.R. Hay
    The origins of the Liberal welfare reforms, 1906–1914

12. H. McLeod
    Religion and the working classes in nineteenth-century Britain

13. J.D. Marshall
    The Old Poor Law 1795–1834: second edition

14. R.J. Morris
    *Class and class consciousness in the industrial revolution,
    1750–1850*

15. P.K. O'Brien
    The economic effects of the American civil war

16. P.L. Payne
    British entrepreneurship in the nineteenth century

17. G.C. Peden
    Keynes, the treasury and British economic policy

18. M.E. Rose
    The relief of poverty, 1834–1914

19. J. Thirsk
    England's agricultural regions and agrarian history, 1500–1750

20. J.R. Ward
    Poverty and progress in the Caribbean, 1800–1960

Economic History Society

The Economic History Society, which numbers around 3,000 members, publishes the *Economic History Review* four times a year (free to members) and holds an annual conference.

Enquiries about membership should be addressed to

The Assistant Secretary
Economic History Society
PO Box 70
Kingswood
Bristol
BS15 5TB

Full-time students may join at special rates.